OWEN HUNTER

Heart Health: Lowering Cholesterol Naturally

First edition

This book was professionally typeset on Reedsy.
Find out more at reedsy.com

Contents

INTRODUCTION

Introduction: A Journey to a Healthier Heart

In today's fast-paced world, where convenience often trumps health, it's easy to lose sight of the importance of maintaining a healthy heart. With heart disease being the leading cause of death worldwide, it's more crucial than ever to take proactive steps towards protecting our cardiovascular well-being. One of the most significant factors contributing to heart disease is high cholesterol levels, a silent threat that can go unnoticed until it's too late.

If you're holding this book in your hands, chances are you or someone you love is looking for natural ways to lower cholesterol and improve overall heart health. Perhaps you've been diagnosed with high cholesterol, or maybe you're simply looking to make positive lifestyle changes to prevent future health problems. Whatever your motivation may be, you've taken the first step towards a healthier, happier life.

The good news is that lowering cholesterol naturally is not only possible but also achievable through simple, yet powerful lifestyle changes. By focusing on nutrition, exercise, stress reduction, and other holistic approaches, you can take control of your heart health and reduce your risk of developing cardiovascular disease.

In "Heart Health: Lowering Cholesterol Naturally," we'll embark on a transformative journey together, exploring the most effective strategies for reducing cholesterol levels without relying solely on medication. This book is designed to empower you with the knowledge and tools you need to make lasting, positive changes in your life.

We'll begin by understanding the fundamentals of cholesterol – what it is, why it matters, and how it affects our bodies. Many people are surprised to learn that not all cholesterol is bad; in fact, our bodies need a certain amount of cholesterol to function properly. We'll delve into the differences between LDL (low-density lipoprotein) and HDL (high-density lipoprotein) cholesterol, and explore the dangers of having high levels of LDL cholesterol in our bloodstream.

Armed with this foundational knowledge, we'll then dive into the power of nutrition and its vital role in managing cholesterol levels. You'll learn about the foods that can help lower cholesterol, as well as those that should be limited or avoided altogether. We'll explore the benefits of plant-based diets, which have been shown to significantly reduce cholesterol levels and improve overall heart health. From fiber-rich fruits and vegetables to heart-healthy fats like olive oil and avocados, you'll discover a world of delicious and nutritious options that can help you achieve your cholesterol goals.

But diet is just one piece of the puzzle. Throughout this book, we'll also examine the importance of regular exercise, stress reduction techniques, and other lifestyle factors that can have a profound impact on your heart health. You'll learn how incorporating physical activity into your daily routine can help raise HDL cholesterol levels, improve circulation, and reduce your risk of heart disease. We'll also explore the link between stress and heart health, and provide practical tips for managing stress through meditation, deep breathing exercises, and other relaxation techniques.

For those interested in exploring supplements as part of their cholesterol-lowering plan, we'll provide an in-depth look at the most popular options available, separating fact from fiction. While some supplements may offer potential benefits, it's crucial to understand their limitations and potential risks, especially when taken without medical supervision. We'll help you navigate the often-confusing world of supplements and provide guidance on when and how to incorporate them into your heart-healthy lifestyle.

Throughout this journey, it's essential to remember that you're not alone. Millions of people worldwide are taking steps to lower their cholesterol and improve their heart health, and their success stories can serve as a source of inspiration and motivation. In this book, we'll share real-life examples of individuals who have transformed their lives through simple, natural changes, proving that it's never too late to start prioritizing your health.

As you embark on this path to a healthier heart, it's important to work closely with your healthcare provider. Regular check-ups and cholesterol screenings can help you monitor your progress and make adjustments to your plan as needed. We'll discuss the importance of partnering with your doctor and provide guidance on when medication may be necessary alongside lifestyle changes.

At the end of the day, lowering cholesterol naturally is about more than just numbers on a chart. It's about taking control of your health, feeling your best, and enjoying a higher quality of life. By making small, sustainable changes to your diet, exercise routine, and overall lifestyle, you can reduce your risk of heart disease and set yourself up for a brighter, healthier future.

In the following chapters, we'll dive deeper into each of these topics, providing you with practical tips, delicious recipes, and expert advice to help you achieve your cholesterol goals. Whether you're just starting on your journey to better heart health or you're looking to take your efforts to the next level, this book will be your guide every step of the way.

So, let's embark on this transformative journey together, armed with the knowledge, tools, and motivation to create lasting, positive change. Your healthier heart awaits!

CHAPTER 1

C hapter 1: Understanding Cholesterol: The Good, the Bad, and the Ugly

Cholesterol is a term that has become synonymous with heart disease, often carrying a negative connotation. However, the truth about cholesterol is much more complex than a simple "good" or "bad" label. To fully grasp the importance of lowering cholesterol naturally, it's essential to understand what cholesterol is, how it functions in our bodies, and why maintaining healthy levels is crucial for our overall well-being.

What is Cholesterol?

Cholesterol is a waxy, fat-like substance that is present in every cell of our bodies. Despite its reputation, cholesterol is essential for various bodily functions. It plays a vital role in the production of hormones, vitamin D, and bile acids that help digest fat. Cholesterol also helps maintain the integrity of our cell membranes, ensuring that they remain stable and function properly.

Our bodies are capable of producing all the cholesterol we need, primarily in the liver. However, we also obtain cholesterol from the foods we eat, particularly animal-based products such as meat, poultry, and dairy. When we consume excessive amounts of dietary cholesterol, or when our bodies produce too much, problems can arise.

The Different Types of Cholesterol

Not all cholesterol is created equal. There are two main types of cholesterol: low-density lipoprotein (LDL) and high-density lipoprotein (HDL). Understanding the difference between these two types is essential for maintaining optimal heart health.

LDL Cholesterol: The "Bad" Cholesterol

LDL cholesterol is often referred to as the "bad" cholesterol. When we have too much LDL cholesterol in our bloodstream, it can slowly build up on the inner walls of our arteries, forming a thick, hard deposit called plaque. Over time, this plaque can narrow or completely block the arteries, reducing blood flow to the heart and other vital organs. This process, known as atherosclerosis, is a major contributor to heart disease, heart attacks, and strokes.

LDL cholesterol is produced naturally by the body, but it can also be increased by consuming foods high in saturated and trans fats, such as fatty meats, full-fat dairy products, and processed snacks. Genetics also play a role in determining an individual's LDL cholesterol levels, with some people inheriting a predisposition to high cholesterol.

HDL Cholesterol: The "Good" Cholesterol

On the other hand, HDL cholesterol is often called the "good" cholesterol. Unlike LDL cholesterol, which contributes to plaque buildup, HDL cholesterol helps remove excess cholesterol from the arteries and transport it back to the liver, where it can be eliminated from the body. In essence, HDL cholesterol acts as a clean-up crew, helping to keep our arteries clear and healthy.

Higher levels of HDL cholesterol are associated with a lower risk of heart disease and stroke. In fact, some studies suggest that for every 1 mg/dL increase in HDL cholesterol, the risk of heart disease decreases by 2-3%. Engaging in regular physical activity, maintaining a healthy weight, and consuming foods rich in monounsaturated and polyunsaturated fats, such as olive oil, nuts, and fatty fish, can help increase HDL cholesterol levels.

Triglycerides: Another Piece of the Puzzle

In addition to LDL and HDL cholesterol, there's another type of fat in the blood called triglycerides. Triglycerides are the most common type of fat in the body, and they are used for energy or stored in fat cells for later use. When we consume more calories than we burn, particularly from carbohydrates, the excess is converted into triglycerides and stored in fat cells.

High levels of triglycerides in the blood have been linked to an increased risk of heart disease and stroke, especially when combined with low HDL cholesterol levels and high LDL cholesterol levels. Factors that can contribute to high triglyceride levels include obesity, physical inactivity, smoking, excessive alcohol consumption, and a diet high in simple sugars and refined carbohydrates.

The Dangers of High Cholesterol

Having high levels of LDL cholesterol and triglycerides in the blood, along with low levels of HDL cholesterol, can have serious consequences for our health. This unhealthy combination, often referred to as "dyslipidemia," is a significant risk factor for cardiovascular disease, the leading cause of death worldwide.

When plaque builds up in the arteries, it can lead to a condition called coronary artery disease (CAD). CAD occurs when the arteries that supply blood to the heart become narrowed or blocked, reducing the flow of oxygen-rich blood to the heart muscle. This can cause chest pain (angina), shortness of breath, and other symptoms. If a plaque ruptures, it can cause a blood clot to form, completely blocking the artery and leading to a heart attack.

High cholesterol can also contribute to the development of peripheral artery disease (PAD), which occurs when the arteries that supply blood to the legs and feet become narrowed or blocked. PAD can cause leg pain, numbness, and weakness, and in severe cases, it can lead to tissue death and amputation.

In addition to its effects on the heart and circulatory system, high cholesterol has been linked to other health problems, such as gallstones and pancreatitis. Gallstones can form when there is too much cholesterol in the bile, leading to painful blockages in the gallbladder. Pancreatitis, an inflammation of the pancreas, can also be caused by high levels of triglycerides in the blood.

The Silent Nature of High Cholesterol

One of the most concerning aspects of high cholesterol is that it often has no symptoms. Many people with high cholesterol feel perfectly healthy, unaware of the damage that is occurring in their arteries. This is why high cholesterol is often referred to as a "silent killer."

The only way to know if you have high cholesterol is to have a blood test called a lipid panel. This test measures your total cholesterol, LDL cholesterol, HDL cholesterol, and triglycerides. The American Heart Association recommends that all adults age 20 and older have their cholesterol checked every four to six years, or more frequently if they have a family history of high cholesterol or other risk factors for heart disease.

If your cholesterol levels are found to be high, your healthcare provider will work with you to develop a plan to lower them. This may include lifestyle changes such as adopting a heart-healthy diet, increasing physical activity, and quitting smoking, as well as medications such as statins, which can help lower LDL cholesterol levels.

The Good News: Lowering Cholesterol Naturally

While high cholesterol can be a serious health concern, the good news is that it is largely preventable and treatable through lifestyle changes. By making simple adjustments to your diet and activity levels, you can significantly reduce your risk of developing high cholesterol and its associated health problems.

In the following chapters, we will explore the most effective strategies for lowering cholesterol naturally, including:

1. Adopting a heart-healthy diet rich in fruits, vegetables, whole grains, and lean proteins
2. Increasing your intake of soluble fiber, which can help reduce LDL cholesterol levels
3. Incorporating healthy fats, such as monounsaturated and polyunsaturated fats, into your diet
4. Engaging in regular physical activity, which can help increase HDL cholesterol levels and reduce triglycerides
5. Maintaining a healthy weight, as excess body fat can contribute to high cholesterol levels
6. Managing stress through relaxation techniques such as meditation and deep breathing exercises
7. Limiting your intake of saturated and trans fats, which can raise LDL cholesterol levels
8. Quitting smoking, which can significantly reduce your risk of heart disease and stroke

By making these lifestyle changes, you can take control of your heart health and reduce your risk of developing high cholesterol and its associated health problems. Remember, it's never too late to start making positive changes in your life, and every small step you take towards a healthier lifestyle can have a significant impact on your overall well-being.

In the next chapter, we will dive deeper into the power of nutrition and explore how eating a heart-healthy diet can help lower cholesterol levels naturally. Get ready to discover a world of delicious, nutritious foods that can help you achieve optimal heart health!

CHAPTER 2

Chapter 2: The Power of Nutrition: Eating Your Way to Lower Cholesterol

When it comes to lowering cholesterol naturally, the power of nutrition cannot be overstated. The foods we eat have a direct impact on our cholesterol levels, and by making strategic choices in our diet, we can significantly reduce our risk of developing heart disease and other health problems associated with high cholesterol.

In this chapter, we will explore the role of diet in managing cholesterol levels, identify the foods that can help lower cholesterol, and provide practical tips for creating a heart-healthy meal plan that is both delicious and nutritious.

The Role of Diet in Managing Cholesterol Levels

The foods we consume play a crucial role in determining our cholesterol levels. When we eat foods that are high in saturated and trans fats, such as fatty meats, full-fat dairy products, and processed snacks, our bodies produce more LDL cholesterol, which can contribute to the buildup of plaque in our arteries.

On the other hand, when we consume foods that are rich in fiber, healthy fats, and nutrient-dense ingredients, we can help lower our LDL cholesterol levels and increase our HDL cholesterol levels, thereby reducing our risk of heart disease and other health problems.

The key to managing cholesterol levels through diet is to focus on consuming a variety of whole, minimally processed foods that are rich in nutrients and low in unhealthy fats. By making simple swaps in our diet, such as replacing saturated fats with unsaturated fats and increasing our intake of fiber-rich foods, we can significantly improve our cholesterol levels and overall heart health.

Foods to Embrace for Lower Cholesterol

When it comes to lowering cholesterol through diet, there are certain foods that should be embraced and consumed regularly. These foods are rich in nutrients that have been shown to have a positive impact on cholesterol levels and heart health. Let's take a closer look at some of the best foods to include in a heart-healthy diet.

1. Fruits and Vegetables

Fruits and vegetables are the foundation of a heart-healthy diet. They are rich in fiber, vitamins, minerals, and antioxidants that can help lower cholesterol levels and reduce inflammation in the body. Aim to consume a variety of colorful fruits and vegetables, such as berries, citrus fruits, leafy greens, and cruciferous vegetables like broccoli and cauliflower.

2. Whole Grains

Whole grains, such as oats, quinoa, brown rice, and whole wheat bread, are an excellent source of fiber and other nutrients that can help lower cholesterol levels. Soluble fiber, in particular, has been shown to reduce LDL cholesterol by binding to it in the digestive tract and preventing its absorption into the bloodstream. Aim to replace refined grains, such as white bread and pasta, with whole-grain alternatives.

3. Legumes

Legumes, such as beans, lentils, and peas, are another excellent source of fiber and plant-based protein. They are also rich in nutrients such as folate, magnesium, and potassium, which can help support heart health. Incorporate legumes into your diet by adding them to soups, salads, and stews, or by using them as a meat alternative in dishes like tacos and chili.

4. Nuts and Seeds

Nuts and seeds, such as almonds, walnuts, chia seeds, and flaxseeds, are rich in healthy fats, fiber, and plant-based protein. They have been shown to help lower LDL cholesterol levels and reduce inflammation in the body. Aim to consume a handful of nuts or a tablespoon of seeds per day as a heart-healthy snack or addition to meals.

5. Fatty Fish

Fatty fish, such as salmon, mackerel, and sardines, are an excellent source of omega-3 fatty acids, which have been shown to have a positive impact on heart health. Omega-3s can help reduce inflammation in the body, lower triglyceride levels, and increase HDL cholesterol levels. Aim to consume fatty fish at least twice per week, or consider taking a high-quality omega-3 supplement if you don't eat fish regularly.

6. Olive Oil

Olive oil is a staple of the Mediterranean diet, which has been associated with a lower risk of heart disease and other chronic health conditions. Olive oil is rich in monounsaturated fats, which can help lower LDL cholesterol levels and increase HDL cholesterol levels. Use olive oil as your primary cooking oil, and drizzle it over salads and vegetables for added flavor and nutrition.

7. Avocados

Avocados are another excellent source of healthy fats, fiber, and nutrients that can support heart health. They are rich in monounsaturated fats, which can help lower LDL cholesterol levels, and they also contain fiber and plant-based compounds that may help reduce inflammation in the body. Incorporate avocados into your diet by adding them to salads, sandwiches, and smoothies, or by using them as a spread on whole-grain toast.

Foods to Avoid for Lower Cholesterol

Just as there are foods that can help lower cholesterol levels, there are also foods that should be limited or avoided altogether in a heart-healthy diet. These foods are typically high in saturated and trans fats, refined carbohydrates, and added sugars, all of which can contribute to high cholesterol levels and other health problems.

1. Saturated and Trans Fats

Saturated and trans fats are two of the most harmful types of fats when it comes to heart health. Saturated fats are found primarily in animal products, such as fatty meats, full-fat dairy products, and tropical oils like coconut and palm oil. Trans fats are found in processed foods that contain partially hydrogenated oils, such as fried foods, baked goods, and snack foods.

Both saturated and trans fats can raise LDL cholesterol levels and increase the risk of heart disease and other health problems. Aim to limit your intake of these unhealthy fats by choosing lean meats, low-fat dairy products, and minimally processed foods.

2. Refined Carbohydrates

Refined carbohydrates, such as white bread, pasta, and sugary snacks, are another type of food that should be limited in a heart-healthy diet. These foods are typically high in calories and low in nutrients, and they can contribute to high blood sugar levels and inflammation in the body.

Instead of consuming refined carbohydrates, choose whole-grain alternatives that are rich in fiber and nutrients. Whole grains can help lower cholesterol levels and reduce the risk of heart disease and other health problems.

3. Added Sugars

Added sugars are another type of food that should be limited in a heart-healthy diet. These sugars are found in a wide variety of processed foods, such as soft drinks, candy, and baked goods, and they can contribute to high triglyceride levels and other health problems.

Aim to limit your intake of added sugars by reading food labels carefully and choosing minimally processed foods that are naturally sweet, such as fruits and vegetables.

Crafting a Heart-Healthy Meal Plan

Now that we've identified the foods that can help lower cholesterol levels and the foods that should be limited or avoided, let's talk about how to craft a heart-healthy meal plan that is both delicious and nutritious.

The key to creating a sustainable heart-healthy meal plan is to focus on variety, balance, and moderation. Aim to include a wide variety of whole, minimally processed foods from each of the major food groups, and be mindful of portion sizes and the balance of nutrients on your plate.

Here are some tips for creating a heart-healthy meal plan:

1. Start with a base of fruits and vegetables. Aim to fill half of your plate with colorful fruits and vegetables at each meal.
2. Choose lean proteins, such as fish, poultry, and plant-based options like legumes and tofu.
3. Incorporate whole grains, such as quinoa, brown rice, and whole-grain bread and pasta.
4. Use healthy fats, such as olive oil, avocado, and nuts and seeds, in moderation.
5. Limit your intake of saturated and trans fats, refined carbohydrates, and added sugars.
6. Drink plenty of water and limit your intake of sugary beverages and alcohol.
7. Practice mindful eating by paying attention to your hunger and fullness cues and eating slowly and without distractions.

Here is an example of a heart-healthy meal plan for one day:

* Breakfast: Oatmeal with berries, chopped nuts, and a drizzle of honey; green tea
    * Snack: Apple slices with almond butter
    * Lunch: Grilled chicken and vegetable salad with a balsamic vinaigrette; whole-grain roll
    * Snack: Carrot sticks and hummus
    * Dinner: Baked salmon with roasted sweet potato and broccoli; quinoa pilaf
    * Dessert: Fresh fruit salad with a dollop of Greek yogurt

Remember, creating a heart-healthy meal plan is not about deprivation or restriction. It's about making small, sustainable changes to your diet that can have a big impact on your cholesterol levels and overall heart health.

Conclusion

The power of nutrition in lowering cholesterol levels cannot be overstated. By focusing on whole, minimally processed foods that are rich in fiber, healthy fats, and nutrients, we can significantly reduce our risk of developing heart disease and other health problems associated with high cholesterol.

Remember, making changes to your diet is not about perfection, but rather about progress. Start by making small, sustainable changes to your eating habits, and gradually work towards creating a heart-healthy meal plan that works for you.

By embracing the foods that can help lower cholesterol levels, such as fruits and vegetables, whole grains, legumes, nuts and seeds, fatty fish, olive oil, and avocados, and limiting your intake of saturated and trans fats, refined carbohydrates, and added sugars, you can take control of your heart health and reduce your risk of developing chronic health conditions.

So, what are you waiting for? Start making changes to your diet today, and experience the power of nutrition in lowering cholesterol levels naturally. Your heart will thank you!

CHAPTER 3

Chapter 3: Unleashing the Potential of Plant-Based Diets

In recent years, plant-based diets have gained significant attention for their numerous health benefits, particularly in the realm of heart health and cholesterol management. A growing body of scientific evidence suggests that adopting a well-planned, plant-based diet can be a powerful tool in lowering cholesterol levels naturally and reducing the risk of cardiovascular disease.

In this chapter, we will explore the science behind plant-based diets and their impact on cholesterol reduction. We will also provide practical tips and strategies for transitioning to a plant-based lifestyle, along with delicious and nutritious recipe ideas to help you get started.

The Science Behind Plant-Based Diets and Cholesterol Reduction

Plant-based diets, which emphasize the consumption of whole, minimally processed foods derived from plants, have been shown to have a significant impact on cholesterol levels and overall heart health. Let's take a closer look at the scientific evidence supporting the use of plant-based diets for cholesterol reduction.

1. Reduced Intake of Saturated and Trans Fats

One of the primary ways in which plant-based diets can help lower cholesterol levels is by reducing the intake of saturated and trans fats. These unhealthy fats, which are found primarily in animal products and processed foods, can raise LDL (bad) cholesterol levels and increase the risk of heart disease.

Plant-based diets, on the other hand, are naturally low in saturated and trans fats, as they emphasize the consumption of whole, minimally processed foods such as fruits, vegetables, whole grains, legumes, nuts, and seeds. By reducing the intake of these unhealthy fats, plant-based diets can help lower LDL cholesterol levels and improve overall heart health.

2. Increased Intake of Fiber

Another key benefit of plant-based diets is their high fiber content. Fiber, particularly soluble fiber, has been shown to have a significant impact on cholesterol levels. Soluble fiber binds to cholesterol in the digestive tract and helps remove it from the body, thereby reducing LDL cholesterol levels.

Plant-based foods such as oats, barley, legumes, fruits, and vegetables are all excellent sources of soluble fiber. By increasing the intake of these fiber-rich foods, plant-based diets can help lower cholesterol levels naturally and improve overall digestive health.

3. Reduced Inflammation

Chronic inflammation is a key contributor to the development of cardiovascular disease, and plant-based diets have been shown to have anti-inflammatory properties. Plant-based foods such as fruits, vegetables, whole grains, and legumes are rich in antioxidants and other anti-inflammatory compounds that can help reduce inflammation in the body.

In contrast, animal-based foods, particularly red and processed meats, have been shown to have pro-inflammatory effects. By reducing the intake of these inflammatory foods and increasing the intake of anti-inflammatory plant-based foods, plant-based diets can help reduce the risk of heart disease and other chronic health conditions.

4. Improved Weight Management

Obesity is a significant risk factor for high cholesterol levels and heart disease, and plant-based diets have been shown to be effective for weight management. Plant-based foods are typically lower in calories and higher in fiber and nutrients than animal-based foods, which can help promote feelings of fullness and reduce overall calorie intake.

In addition, plant-based diets have been shown to increase the body's sensitivity to insulin, a hormone that helps regulate blood sugar levels and promote weight loss. By improving insulin sensitivity and promoting weight loss, plant-based diets can help lower cholesterol levels and reduce the risk of heart disease.

Transitioning to a Plant-Based Lifestyle

While the benefits of plant-based diets for cholesterol reduction are clear, transitioning to a plant-based lifestyle can be challenging for some individuals. Here are some practical tips and strategies for making the transition:

1. Start Small

If you are new to plant-based eating, it's important to start small and make gradual changes to your diet over time. Consider incorporating one or two plant-based meals into your diet each week, and gradually increase the frequency as you become more comfortable with the lifestyle.

2. Focus on Whole, Minimally Processed Foods

When transitioning to a plant-based diet, it's important to focus on whole, minimally processed foods such as fruits, vegetables, whole grains, legumes, nuts, and seeds. These foods are rich in nutrients and fiber and can help promote feelings of fullness and satisfaction.

3. Experiment with New Foods and Flavors

One of the joys of plant-based eating is the opportunity to explore new foods and flavors. Don't be afraid to experiment with new ingredients and recipes, and seek out plant-based versions of your favorite dishes.

4. Plan Ahead

Planning ahead is key to success when transitioning to a plant-based lifestyle. Take the time to plan your meals and snacks for the week, and make sure you have plenty of plant-based options on hand. Consider batch cooking and meal prepping to save time and ensure that you always have healthy options available.

5. Seek Support

Transitioning to a plant-based lifestyle can be challenging, especially if you are doing it alone. Consider seeking support from friends, family members, or a registered dietitian who can provide guidance and encouragement along the way.

Delicious and Nutritious Plant-Based Recipes

One of the best ways to embrace a plant-based lifestyle is to experiment with delicious and nutritious recipes that showcase the versatility and flavor of plant-based ingredients. Here are a few recipe ideas to get you started:

1. Breakfast: Overnight Oats with Fresh Berries and Chia Seeds
   Ingredients:
   - 1/2 cup rolled oats
   - 1/2 cup unsweetened almond milk
   - 1/4 cup fresh berries (such as strawberries, blueberries, or raspberries)
   - 1 tablespoon chia seeds
   - 1/2 teaspoon vanilla extract
   - Pinch of cinnamon

Instructions:

1. In a jar or container with a lid, combine the rolled oats, almond milk, chia seeds, vanilla extract, and cinnamon. Stir well to combine.

2. Place the lid on the jar and refrigerate overnight, or for at least 4 hours.

3. In the morning, remove the lid and stir the oats. Top with fresh berries and enjoy!

2. Lunch: Chickpea and Avocado Salad Sandwich

Ingredients:

- 1 can (15 ounces) chickpeas, drained and rinsed
- 1 ripe avocado, mashed
- 1/4 cup diced red onion
- 1/4 cup chopped fresh cilantro
- 1 tablespoon lime juice
- Salt and pepper to taste
- 4 slices whole-grain bread
- Sliced tomato and lettuce for serving

Instructions:

1. In a bowl, combine the chickpeas, mashed avocado, red onion, cilantro, and lime juice. Mash the mixture with a fork until well combined. Season with salt and pepper to taste.

2. Toast the bread slices until golden brown.

3. Spread the chickpea and avocado mixture evenly over two of the bread slices. Top with sliced tomato and lettuce, and cover with the remaining bread slices.

4. Cut the sandwiches in half and serve immediately.

3. Dinner: Quinoa and Black Bean Burrito Bowls

Ingredients:

- 1 cup uncooked quinoa, rinsed
- 2 cups water
- 1 can (15 ounces) black beans, drained and rinsed

- 1 red bell pepper, diced
- 1/2 red onion, diced
- 1/2 cup corn kernels (fresh, frozen, or canned)
- 1/4 cup chopped fresh cilantro
- 1 lime, juiced
- 1 tablespoon olive oil
- 1 teaspoon ground cumin
- Salt and pepper to taste
- Optional toppings: diced avocado, salsa, and shredded lettuce

Instructions:

1. In a medium saucepan, combine the quinoa and water. Bring to a boil, then reduce heat to low, cover, and simmer for 15 minutes, or until the quinoa is tender and the water is absorbed.
2. In a large bowl, combine the cooked quinoa, black beans, bell pepper, onion, corn, and cilantro.
3. In a small bowl, whisk together the lime juice, olive oil, cumin, salt, and pepper.
4. Pour the dressing over the quinoa mixture and stir to combine.
5. Divide the quinoa mixture evenly among four bowls. Top with diced avocado, salsa, and shredded lettuce, if desired.

Conclusion

The potential of plant-based diets for lowering cholesterol levels naturally and improving overall heart health is truly remarkable. By reducing the intake of saturated and trans fats, increasing the intake of fiber, reducing inflammation, and promoting weight loss, plant-based diets can help individuals achieve their cholesterol goals and reduce their risk of cardiovascular disease.

While transitioning to a plant-based lifestyle can be challenging, it is a journey worth taking for the sake of your health and well-being. By starting small, focusing on whole, minimally processed foods, experimenting with new flavors and recipes, planning ahead, and seeking support, you can successfully embrace a plant-based lifestyle and reap the many benefits it has to offer.

Remember, the key to success with plant-based eating is to focus on progress, not perfection. Every small step you take towards a more plant-based diet is a step in the right direction for your health and the health of the planet.

So why not give plant-based eating a try? With a little creativity and an open mind, you may be surprised at how delicious, satisfying, and beneficial a plant-based diet can be. Your heart (and your taste buds) will thank you!

CHAPTER 4

Chapter 4: The Fiber Factor: Navigating the Path to Heart Health

Fiber is an essential component of a heart-healthy diet, playing a crucial role in managing cholesterol levels and promoting overall cardiovascular well-being. Despite its importance, many people fall short of consuming the recommended daily intake of fiber, missing out on its numerous health benefits.

In this chapter, we will delve into the world of dietary fiber, exploring its various types, sources, and mechanisms of action in the body. We will also provide practical tips and strategies for incorporating more fiber-rich foods into your daily routine, making it easier than ever to harness the power of this essential nutrient for optimal heart health.

Understanding the Importance of Dietary Fiber

Dietary fiber is a type of carbohydrate that is not digested or absorbed by the body. Instead, it passes through the digestive system relatively intact, providing a range of health benefits along the way.

There are two main types of dietary fiber: soluble and insoluble. Both types are important for overall health, but they differ in their properties and effects on the body.

Soluble Fiber

Soluble fiber dissolves in water to form a gel-like substance. This type of fiber is known for its cholesterol-lowering properties, as it binds to cholesterol in the digestive tract and helps remove it from the body. Soluble fiber is found in foods such as oats, barley, legumes, fruits, and vegetables.

The mechanisms by which soluble fiber lowers cholesterol are complex and multifaceted. One key mechanism involves the binding of bile acids in the digestive tract. Bile acids are produced by the liver and are necessary for the digestion and absorption of fats. When soluble fiber binds to bile acids, it prevents their reabsorption and promotes their excretion from the body. As a result, the liver must produce more bile acids to replace those that have been lost, using up cholesterol in the process. This leads to a reduction in circulating cholesterol levels over time.

In addition to its bile acid-binding properties, soluble fiber also helps regulate blood sugar levels by slowing the absorption of glucose in the digestive tract. This can be particularly beneficial for individuals with diabetes or prediabetes, as it helps prevent rapid spikes and crashes in blood sugar levels.

Insoluble Fiber
Insoluble fiber, on the other hand, does not dissolve in water and remains largely intact as it passes through the digestive system. This type of fiber is known for its ability to promote regular bowel movements and prevent constipation. Insoluble fiber is found in foods such as whole grains, nuts, seeds, and the skins of fruits and vegetables.

While insoluble fiber does not have a direct impact on cholesterol levels, it is still an important component of a heart-healthy diet. By promoting regular bowel movements and preventing constipation, insoluble fiber helps reduce the risk of hemorrhoids, diverticular disease, and other digestive disorders. It also helps promote feelings of fullness and satiety, which can be beneficial for weight management.

The Benefits of a High-Fiber Diet

Consuming a diet rich in both soluble and insoluble fiber has been shown to provide a range of health benefits, particularly in the realm of heart health. Some of the key benefits of a high-fiber diet include:

1. Lower Cholesterol Levels

As mentioned earlier, soluble fiber helps lower cholesterol levels by binding to bile acids in the digestive tract and promoting their excretion from the body. Studies have shown that consuming just 5-10 grams of soluble fiber per day can reduce LDL (bad) cholesterol levels by as much as 5%.

2. Reduced Risk of Heart Disease

In addition to lowering cholesterol levels, a high-fiber diet has been shown to reduce the risk of heart disease by a variety of other mechanisms. For example, fiber helps reduce inflammation in the body, which is a key contributor to the development of atherosclerosis and other cardiovascular disorders. Fiber also helps lower blood pressure and improve insulin sensitivity, both of which are important for maintaining a healthy heart.

3. Better Weight Management

Fiber-rich foods tend to be more filling and satisfying than low-fiber foods, which can help with weight management. When you feel full and satisfied after a meal, you are less likely to overeat or snack on unhealthy foods later in the day. In addition, fiber helps slow the absorption of glucose in the digestive tract, which can help regulate blood sugar levels and prevent rapid spikes and crashes that can lead to overeating.

4. Improved Digestive Health

As mentioned earlier, insoluble fiber helps promote regular bowel movements and prevent constipation. This can help reduce the risk of hemorrhoids, diverticular disease, and other digestive disorders. In addition, fiber acts as a prebiotic, feeding the beneficial bacteria in the gut and promoting a healthy gut microbiome.

5. Reduced Risk of Other Chronic Diseases

In addition to its benefits for heart health, a high-fiber diet has been shown to reduce the risk of other chronic diseases such as type 2 diabetes, certain types of cancer, and obesity. This is likely due to the many protective properties of fiber, including its ability to reduce inflammation, regulate blood sugar levels, and promote feelings of fullness and satiety.

Incorporating More Fiber into Your Diet

Now that we have explored the many benefits of a high-fiber diet, let's talk about how to incorporate more fiber-rich foods into your daily routine. Here are some practical tips and strategies to get you started:

1. Choose Whole Grains

One of the easiest ways to boost your fiber intake is to choose whole grains over refined grains whenever possible. Look for breads, pastas, and cereals that list a whole grain as the first ingredient, such as whole wheat, oats, or quinoa. Aim for at least 3 servings of whole grains per day.

2. Eat More Fruits and Vegetables

Fruits and vegetables are excellent sources of both soluble and insoluble fiber, as well as a range of other essential nutrients. Aim for at least 5 servings of fruits and vegetables per day, choosing a variety of colors and types to ensure that you are getting a diverse range of nutrients.

3. Incorporate Legumes

Legumes, such as beans, lentils, and peas, are some of the best sources of soluble fiber. They are also an excellent source of plant-based protein and other essential nutrients. Try incorporating legumes into your diet at least 2-3 times per week, either as a main dish or as a side.

4. Snack on Nuts and Seeds

Nuts and seeds are another great source of fiber, as well as healthy fats and other essential nutrients. Choose raw or dry-roasted nuts and seeds, and aim for a serving size of about 1 ounce (or a small handful) per day.

5. Use Fiber Supplements

If you are having trouble meeting your daily fiber needs through food alone, you may want to consider using a fiber supplement. There are many different types of fiber supplements available, including psyllium husk, methylcellulose, and inulin. Talk to your healthcare provider or registered dietitian to determine which type of supplement may be right for you.

6. Read Nutrition Labels

When grocery shopping, be sure to read nutrition labels carefully to identify foods that are high in fiber. Look for foods that contain at least 3 grams of fiber per serving, and aim for a total daily intake of at least 25-38 grams of fiber per day.

7. Experiment with New Recipes

Finally, don't be afraid to experiment with new recipes and ingredients that are high in fiber. There are countless delicious and nutritious recipes available online and in cookbooks that feature fiber-rich foods such as whole grains, legumes, fruits, and vegetables. Try incorporating one new high-fiber recipe into your meal plan each week to keep things interesting and enjoyable.

Conclusion

The fiber factor is a critical component of any heart-healthy diet, playing a vital role in managing cholesterol levels, promoting digestive health, and reducing the risk of various chronic diseases. By understanding the different types of fiber and their unique properties, as well as incorporating a variety of fiber-rich foods into your daily routine, you can take a proactive approach to optimizing your cardiovascular well-being.

Remember, the key to success with any dietary change is to start small and make gradual, sustainable shifts over time. Don't try to overhaul your entire diet overnight, but rather focus on making one or two small changes each week until they become a natural part of your routine.

Whether you are just starting on your journey to better heart health or are looking to take your fiber intake to the next level, the tips and strategies outlined in this chapter can help you navigate the path to success. So go ahead and embrace the fiber factor – your heart (and your taste buds) will thank you!

CHAPTER 5

Chapter 5: Harnessing the Power of Omega-3 Fatty Acids

When it comes to promoting heart health and lowering cholesterol levels naturally, few nutrients have garnered as much attention in recent years as omega-3 fatty acids. These essential fatty acids, found primarily in fatty fish and certain plant-based sources, have been shown to provide a wide range of cardiovascular benefits, from reducing inflammation and blood clotting to improving the health of our blood vessels and cell membranes.

In this chapter, we will take a deep dive into the world of omega-3 fatty acids, exploring their unique properties, the various food sources available, and the ways in which they can help support optimal heart health. We will also discuss the importance of balancing omega-3 intake with that of another essential fatty acid, omega-6, in order to maintain a healthy ratio and maximize the benefits of both.

The Role of Omega-3s in Promoting Heart Health

Omega-3 fatty acids are a type of polyunsaturated fat that is essential for human health. Unlike other types of fat, such as saturated and monounsaturated fats, our bodies cannot produce omega-3s on their own, which means we must obtain them through our diet.

There are three main types of omega-3 fatty acids: eicosapentaenoic acid

(EPA), docosahexaenoic acid (DHA), and alpha-linolenic acid (ALA). EPA and DHA are found primarily in fatty fish, such as salmon, mackerel, and sardines, while ALA is found in plant-based sources such as flaxseed, chia seeds, and walnuts.

The cardiovascular benefits of omega-3s are numerous and well-documented. Here are just a few of the ways in which these essential fatty acids can help promote heart health:

1. Reducing Inflammation

Chronic inflammation is a major contributor to the development of cardiovascular disease, as it can damage the lining of our blood vessels and contribute to the formation of atherosclerotic plaques. Omega-3 fatty acids have been shown to have potent anti-inflammatory properties, helping to reduce inflammation throughout the body and protect against cardiovascular damage.

2. Lowering Triglycerides

Triglycerides are a type of fat that circulates in the bloodstream and can contribute to the development of heart disease when levels become too high. Omega-3 fatty acids, particularly EPA and DHA, have been shown to significantly reduce triglyceride levels in the blood, thereby lowering the risk of cardiovascular disease.

3. Reducing Blood Clotting

Blood clots can be a major risk factor for heart attack and stroke, as they can block the flow of blood to the heart or brain. Omega-3 fatty acids have been shown to reduce the tendency of blood to clot, thereby reducing the risk of these serious cardiovascular events.

4. Improving Endothelial Function

The endothelium is the inner lining of our blood vessels, and its health is critical for maintaining proper blood flow and preventing the development of atherosclerosis. Omega-3 fatty acids have been shown to improve endothelial function by increasing the production of nitric oxide, a compound that helps to relax and widen blood vessels.

5. Reducing Blood Pressure

High blood pressure, or hypertension, is a major risk factor for heart disease and stroke. Omega-3 fatty acids have been shown to help reduce blood pressure by improving the elasticity of blood vessels and reducing the resistance to blood flow.

Best Sources of Omega-3 Fatty Acids

Now that we have explored some of the key cardiovascular benefits of omega-3 fatty acids, let's take a closer look at the best dietary sources of these essential nutrients.

Fatty Fish

As mentioned earlier, fatty fish are one of the best sources of EPA and DHA, the two most potent forms of omega-3 fatty acids. Some of the best fish sources of omega-3s include:

- Salmon
  - Mackerel
  - Sardines
  - Anchovies
  - Herring
  - Tuna (particularly albacore and bluefin)

When choosing fish, it is important to consider both the omega-3 content and the potential for contaminants such as mercury. Smaller, cold-water fish such as sardines and anchovies tend to have lower levels of contaminants and higher levels of omega-3s compared to larger, predatory fish like tuna and swordfish.

Plant-Based Sources

While EPA and DHA are found primarily in fatty fish, ALA is found in a variety of plant-based sources, including:

- Flaxseed and flaxseed oil
    - Chia seeds
    - Hemp seeds
    - Walnuts
    - Soybeans and soybean oil
    - Canola oil

It is important to note that while ALA is an essential omega-3 fatty acid, it must be converted by the body into EPA and DHA in order to provide the same cardiovascular benefits. This conversion process is relatively inefficient in humans, with only a small percentage of ALA being converted into EPA and DHA. For this reason, it is generally recommended to obtain EPA and DHA directly from fatty fish or fish oil supplements, rather than relying solely on plant-based sources of ALA.

Omega-3 Supplements

For individuals who do not consume fatty fish regularly or who have difficulty obtaining enough omega-3s through diet alone, omega-3 supplements can be a useful option. These supplements typically come in the form of fish oil capsules or liquids, and contain concentrated doses of EPA and DHA.

When choosing an omega-3 supplement, it is important to look for a high-quality product that has been purified to remove contaminants such as mercury and PCBs. It is also important to choose a supplement that contains a balanced ratio of EPA and DHA, as both of these fatty acids have unique cardiovascular benefits.

As with any supplement, it is always best to consult with a healthcare provider before starting an omega-3 regimen, particularly if you have any pre-existing health conditions or are taking medications that may interact with omega-3s.

Balancing Omega-3 and Omega-6 Intake

While omega-3 fatty acids are essential for heart health, it is important to consider their intake in the context of another essential fatty acid: omega-6. Omega-6 fatty acids, found primarily in vegetable oils and processed foods, are also important for human health, but they can have pro-inflammatory effects when consumed in excess.

In the modern Western diet, the ratio of omega-6 to omega-3 fatty acids has become increasingly skewed, with many people consuming far more omega-6s than omega-3s. This imbalance has been linked to an increased risk of chronic diseases such as heart disease, diabetes, and certain cancers.

To help maintain a healthy balance of omega-3 and omega-6 fatty acids, it is important to:

1. Increase intake of omega-3-rich foods such as fatty fish and plant-based sources of ALA.
2. Reduce intake of processed foods and vegetable oils high in omega-6s, such as soybean, corn, and sunflower oils.
3. Choose healthy, whole-food sources of both omega-3s and omega-6s, such as nuts, seeds, and avocados.
4. Consider using omega-3 supplements if necessary to achieve a balanced intake.

By focusing on a balanced intake of both omega-3 and omega-6 fatty acids, we can help optimize the cardiovascular benefits of these essential nutrients and promote overall health and well-being.

Conclusion

The power of omega-3 fatty acids in promoting heart health and lowering cholesterol levels naturally cannot be overstated. By incorporating a variety of omega-3-rich foods into our diets, such as fatty fish and plant-based sources of ALA, we can help reduce inflammation, lower triglycerides, improve endothelial function, and reduce the risk of serious cardiovascular events such as heart attack and stroke.

At the same time, it is important to consider the balance of omega-3 and omega-6 fatty acids in our diets, and to strive for a more balanced intake that promotes overall health and well-being. By making small, sustainable changes to our diets and lifestyles, we can harness the power of these essential nutrients and take a proactive approach to optimizing our cardiovascular health.

Whether you are just starting on your journey to better heart health or are looking to take your omega-3 intake to the next level, the tips and strategies outlined in this chapter can help guide you on your path to success. So go ahead and embrace the power of omega-3s – your heart (and your taste buds) will thank you!

CHAPTER 6

Chapter 6: Phytosterols: Nature's Secret Weapon Against Cholesterol

In the quest for natural ways to lower cholesterol and promote heart health, one group of compounds has emerged as a promising ally: phytosterols. Found naturally in a variety of plant-based foods, phytosterols have been shown to have potent cholesterol-lowering properties, making them an intriguing option for those looking to manage their cholesterol levels through dietary means.

In this chapter, we will explore the world of phytosterols, delving into their unique mechanisms of action, the various food sources available, and the potential benefits and drawbacks of phytosterol supplements. By the end of this chapter, you will have a comprehensive understanding of how these powerful plant compounds can fit into a heart-healthy lifestyle and help you achieve your cholesterol management goals.

What are Phytosterols, and How Do They Work?

Phytosterols, also known as plant sterols, are a group of compounds found naturally in the cell membranes of plants. Structurally similar to cholesterol, phytosterols play a vital role in maintaining the integrity and fluidity of plant cell membranes, just as cholesterol does in animal cells.

There are several different types of phytosterols, including beta-sitosterol, campesterol, and stigmasterol, each with slightly different chemical structures and properties. However, all phytosterols share a common mechanism of action when it comes to lowering cholesterol levels in the human body.

When we consume phytosterols, they are absorbed into the intestinal cells, where they compete with cholesterol for incorporation into mixed micelles, the tiny droplets of lipids that are formed during digestion. Because phytosterols are more hydrophobic (water-repelling) than cholesterol, they are preferentially incorporated into the micelles, displacing cholesterol in the process.

As a result, less cholesterol is absorbed from the intestine into the bloodstream, and more is excreted in the feces. Over time, this can lead to a significant reduction in total and LDL (bad) cholesterol levels, without affecting HDL (good) cholesterol levels.

In addition to their cholesterol-lowering effects, phytosterols have also been shown to have anti-inflammatory and antioxidant properties, which may help to reduce the risk of cardiovascular disease and other chronic health conditions.

Foods Rich in Phytosterols

Phytosterols are found naturally in a wide variety of plant-based foods, including:

1. Vegetable Oils

Vegetable oils are one of the richest sources of phytosterols, with particularly high levels found in rice bran oil, wheat germ oil, and corn oil. Other vegetable oils that contain significant amounts of phytosterols include canola oil, soybean oil, and sesame oil.

2. Nuts and Seeds

Nuts and seeds are another excellent source of phytosterols, with particularly high levels found in pistachios, sunflower seeds, and sesame seeds. Other nut and seed sources of phytosterols include almonds, cashews, and pumpkin seeds.

3. Whole Grains

Whole grains, such as wheat, oats, and barley, are also good sources of phytosterols. In particular, wheat germ and bran are particularly rich in these plant compounds.

4. Legumes

Legumes, such as beans, lentils, and peas, are another good source of phytosterols. In particular, soybeans and soy-based products, such as tofu and tempeh, are rich in these cholesterol-lowering compounds.

5. Fruits and Vegetables

While fruits and vegetables are not as rich in phytosterols as some other plant-based foods, they still contain significant amounts of these beneficial compounds. Some of the best fruit and vegetable sources of phytosterols include avocados, berries, and dark leafy greens such as spinach and kale.

It is worth noting that while phytosterols are found naturally in a wide variety of plant-based foods, the amounts present in these foods may not be sufficient to have a significant impact on cholesterol levels when consumed as part of a typical diet. For this reason, many people turn to phytosterol supplements or fortified foods as a way to boost their intake of these beneficial compounds.

Phytosterol Supplements: Are They Worth It?

In recent years, phytosterol supplements have become increasingly popular as a natural way to lower cholesterol levels and promote heart health. These supplements typically come in the form of capsules or tablets and contain concentrated doses of phytosterols derived from vegetable oils or other plant-based sources.

Studies have shown that phytosterol supplements can be effective in reducing total and LDL cholesterol levels when taken in doses of 1-3 grams per day. In fact, the FDA has approved a health claim for phytosterol supplements, stating that "foods containing at least 0.65 gram per serving of vegetable oil plant sterol esters, eaten twice a day with meals for a daily total intake of at least 1.3 grams, as part of a diet low in saturated fat and cholesterol, may reduce the risk of heart disease."

However, as with any supplement, there are potential drawbacks and considerations to keep in mind when it comes to phytosterol supplements. Here are a few key points to consider:

1. Potential for Nutrient Interactions

Phytosterols can interfere with the absorption of certain fat-soluble vitamins, such as vitamin A, D, E, and K. While this effect is generally modest and unlikely to cause deficiencies in most people, it is something to be aware of, particularly for those with pre-existing nutrient deficiencies or those taking medications that may interact with fat-soluble vitamins.

2. Quality and Purity Concerns

As with any supplement, it is important to choose a high-quality, reputable brand of phytosterol supplement to ensure purity and potency. Some lower-quality supplements may contain contaminants or fillers that can reduce their effectiveness or even pose health risks.

3. Cost Considerations

Phytosterol supplements can be relatively expensive compared to other cholesterol-lowering options, such as dietary changes or prescription medications. While they may be a worthwhile investment for some people, it is important to consider the cost in the context of your overall health goals and budget.

4. Importance of a Comprehensive Approach

While phytosterol supplements can be a useful tool in the fight against high cholesterol, it is important to remember that they are not a magic bullet. To truly optimize heart health and reduce the risk of cardiovascular disease, it is important to take a comprehensive approach that includes a healthy diet, regular exercise, stress management, and other lifestyle factors.

If you are considering taking phytosterol supplements to lower your cholesterol levels, it is always best to consult with a healthcare provider first. They can help you weigh the potential benefits and risks, determine an appropriate dosage, and monitor your response to the supplement over time.

The Bottom Line on Phytosterols and Heart Health

Phytosterols are a fascinating and promising group of compounds when it comes to natural approaches to lowering cholesterol and promoting heart health. By competing with cholesterol for absorption in the intestine, phytosterols can help to reduce total and LDL cholesterol levels, without affecting HDL cholesterol or posing significant side effects.

While phytosterols are found naturally in a variety of plant-based foods, including vegetable oils, nuts and seeds, whole grains, legumes, and certain fruits and vegetables, the amounts present in these foods may not be sufficient to have a significant impact on cholesterol levels when consumed as part of a typical diet. For this reason, many people turn to phytosterol supplements or fortified foods as a way to boost their intake of these beneficial compounds.

However, as with any supplement or dietary approach, it is important to take a comprehensive and individualized approach to heart health, one that takes into account a variety of lifestyle factors and personal health goals. By working closely with a healthcare provider and making informed decisions about phytosterol intake, you can harness the power of these natural compounds to support your cholesterol management goals and promote overall cardiovascular well-being.

So, whether you choose to incorporate more phytosterol-rich foods into your diet, consider a phytosterol supplement, or simply focus on other heart-healthy lifestyle habits, remember that every step you take towards better cardiovascular health is a step in the right direction. With a little knowledge, commitment, and perseverance, you can unlock the potential of phytosterols and other natural approaches to create a stronger, healthier heart for years to come.

CHAPTER 7

Chapter 7: The Antioxidant Arsenal: Fighting Cholesterol with Superfoods

In the ongoing battle against high cholesterol and cardiovascular disease, there is one group of nutrients that has emerged as a powerful ally: antioxidants. Found in a wide variety of colorful, plant-based foods, antioxidants have been shown to have potent cholesterol-lowering and heart-protective properties, making them a vital component of any heart-healthy diet.

In this chapter, we will explore the fascinating world of antioxidants, delving into their unique mechanisms of action, the various food sources available, and the ways in which they can be incorporated into a delicious and nutritious diet. By the end of this chapter, you will have a comprehensive understanding of how these superhero nutrients can help you optimize your cholesterol levels, reduce your risk of heart disease, and unlock a new level of vitality and wellness.

The Link Between Antioxidants and Heart Health

Antioxidants are a diverse group of compounds that share a common ability to neutralize harmful molecules known as free radicals. Free radicals are unstable molecules that are produced naturally in the body as a byproduct of cellular metabolism, as well as through exposure to environmental toxins such as pollution, radiation, and cigarette smoke.

When left unchecked, free radicals can damage cells, proteins, and DNA, leading to a state of oxidative stress that has been linked to a wide range of chronic diseases, including heart disease, cancer, and neurological disorders. Antioxidants work by donating an electron to the free radical, stabilizing it and preventing it from causing further damage.

In the context of heart health, antioxidants have been shown to have a number of important benefits, including:

1. Reducing LDL Oxidation

One of the key ways in which antioxidants protect against heart disease is by reducing the oxidation of LDL (bad) cholesterol. When LDL cholesterol becomes oxidized, it is more likely to stick to the walls of the arteries and contribute to the formation of atherosclerotic plaques. Antioxidants help to prevent this oxidation, reducing the risk of plaque formation and improving overall cardiovascular health.

2. Improving Endothelial Function

The endothelium is the inner lining of the blood vessels, and its health is critical for maintaining proper blood flow and preventing the development of atherosclerosis. Antioxidants have been shown to improve endothelial function by reducing inflammation and promoting the production of nitric oxide, a compound that helps to relax and widen the blood vessels.

3. Reducing Inflammation

Chronic inflammation is a major contributor to the development of cardiovascular disease, as well as many other chronic health conditions. Antioxidants have powerful anti-inflammatory properties, helping to reduce inflammation throughout the body and protect against the damaging effects of oxidative stress.

4. Supporting Healthy Cholesterol Levels

While the primary focus of antioxidants is on reducing oxidative stress and inflammation, some antioxidants have also been shown to have direct cholesterol-lowering effects. For example, the antioxidant compound resveratrol, found in red wine and certain fruits, has been shown to inhibit the production of LDL cholesterol in the liver, while the antioxidant lycopene, found in tomatoes and other red fruits and vegetables, has been shown to reduce total and LDL cholesterol levels.

Top Antioxidant-Rich Superfoods to Include in Your Diet

Now that we have a better understanding of the link between antioxidants and heart health, let's take a closer look at some of the top antioxidant-rich superfoods that you can easily incorporate into your diet for maximum benefit.

1. Berries

Berries, including blueberries, strawberries, raspberries, and blackberries, are some of the most antioxidant-rich foods on the planet. They are particularly high in a type of antioxidant called anthocyanins, which give berries their vibrant red, blue, and purple colors. Studies have shown that regular consumption of berries can help to reduce inflammation, improve endothelial function, and lower the risk of heart disease.

2. Dark Leafy Greens

Dark leafy greens, such as spinach, kale, and Swiss chard, are another excellent source of antioxidants. They are particularly high in a type of antioxidant called lutein, which has been shown to reduce inflammation and improve cardiovascular health. Dark leafy greens are also rich in other heart-healthy nutrients, such as folate, magnesium, and vitamin K.

3. Nuts and Seeds

Nuts and seeds, such as almonds, walnuts, chia seeds, and flaxseeds, are rich in antioxidants as well as healthy fats, fiber, and plant-based protein. They are particularly high in a type of antioxidant called vitamin E, which has been shown to reduce inflammation and improve endothelial function.

Studies have also shown that regular consumption of nuts and seeds can help to lower total and LDL cholesterol levels.

4. Dark Chocolate

Dark chocolate, particularly varieties with a high cocoa content (70% or higher), is an excellent source of antioxidants. It is particularly high in a type of antioxidant called flavonoids, which have been shown to reduce inflammation, improve endothelial function, and lower the risk of heart disease. However, it is important to choose dark chocolate in moderation, as it is also high in calories and sugar.

5. Red Wine

Red wine, particularly varieties made from Pinot Noir or Cabernet Sauvignon grapes, is another excellent source of antioxidants. It is particularly high in a type of antioxidant called resveratrol, which has been shown to have potent anti-inflammatory and cholesterol-lowering effects. However, it is important to consume red wine in moderation, as excessive alcohol intake can have negative effects on heart health.

6. Citrus Fruits

Citrus fruits, such as oranges, grapefruits, and lemons, are rich in a type of antioxidant called vitamin C. Vitamin C has been shown to reduce inflammation, improve endothelial function, and boost the immune system. Citrus fruits are also a good source of other heart-healthy nutrients, such as folate and potassium.

7. Tomatoes

Tomatoes, particularly cooked or processed varieties such as tomato sauce and paste, are an excellent source of the antioxidant lycopene. Lycopene has been shown to reduce inflammation, improve endothelial function, and lower total and LDL cholesterol levels. Tomatoes are also a good source of other heart-healthy nutrients, such as vitamin C and potassium.

Maximizing the Benefits of Antioxidants

While incorporating more antioxidant-rich foods into your diet is an excellent way to support heart health and lower cholesterol levels, there are a few key strategies that can help you maximize the benefits of these powerful nutrients:

1. Eat a Rainbow

One of the easiest ways to ensure that you are getting a wide variety of antioxidants in your diet is to eat a rainbow of colorful fruits and vegetables. Each color represents a different type of antioxidant, so by eating a variety of colors, you can ensure that you are getting a broad spectrum of heart-healthy nutrients.

2. Cook Smart

While some antioxidants, such as vitamin C, are heat-sensitive and can be degraded by cooking, others, such as lycopene, are actually enhanced by cooking. To maximize the antioxidant content of your meals, try to include a mix of raw and cooked fruits and vegetables, and opt for gentler cooking methods such as steaming or sautéing over high-heat methods like frying or grilling.

3. Pair Wisely

Some antioxidants, such as vitamin C and vitamin E, work together synergistically to provide even greater heart-health benefits. To maximize these synergistic effects, try pairing antioxidant-rich foods together, such as combining citrus fruits with nuts or seeds, or adding diced tomatoes to your dark leafy green salads.

4. Supplement Smartly

While it is always best to get your antioxidants from whole food sources, some people may benefit from antioxidant supplements, particularly if they have trouble meeting their needs through diet alone. However, it is important to choose high-quality supplements from reputable brands, and to always consult with a healthcare provider before starting any new supplement regimen.

The Power of Antioxidants: A Final Word

Antioxidants are a powerful tool in the fight against high cholesterol and cardiovascular disease, and incorporating more of these superhero nutrients into your diet can have a profound impact on your overall health and well-being.

By focusing on colorful, plant-based foods such as berries, dark leafy greens, nuts and seeds, dark chocolate, red wine, citrus fruits, and tomatoes, you can easily boost your intake of heart-healthy antioxidants and start reaping the benefits of these powerful compounds.

Remember, the key to success with any dietary change is to start small and build gradually over time. Don't try to overhaul your entire diet overnight, but rather focus on making one or two small changes each week, such as swapping out your usual snack for a handful of antioxidant-rich berries or adding a side of sautéed spinach to your evening meal.

As you continue to incorporate more antioxidant-rich foods into your diet, you may start to notice improvements in your energy levels, your digestion, and your overall sense of well-being. And over time, these small changes can add up to big benefits for your heart health, your cholesterol levels, and your overall vitality and resilience.

So why wait? Start harnessing the power of antioxidants today, and discover just how delicious and nutritious the path to better heart health can be!

CHAPTER 8

C hapter 8: Spices and Herbs: Flavorful Allies in the Battle Against Cholesterol

When it comes to lowering cholesterol and promoting heart health, many people focus solely on the macronutrients in their diet, such as fats, proteins, and carbohydrates. However, there is another category of nutrients that can have a profound impact on cardiovascular health: spices and herbs.

These flavorful ingredients, which have been used for centuries in traditional medicine systems around the world, are not only packed with antioxidants and other beneficial compounds, but they can also add depth, complexity, and satisfaction to even the simplest of meals.

In this chapter, we will explore the fascinating world of spices and herbs, delving into the specific compounds and mechanisms that give them their cholesterol-lowering properties. We will also share some practical tips and recipes for incorporating more of these flavorful allies into your daily diet, so you can start reaping the benefits of their heart-healthy powers today.

Exploring the Cholesterol-Lowering Properties of Spices and Herbs

Spices and herbs are not just flavorful additions to your favorite dishes; they are also potent sources of antioxidants, anti-inflammatory compounds, and other beneficial nutrients that can help lower cholesterol levels and protect against heart disease.

Here are just a few of the ways in which spices and herbs can support cardiovascular health:

1. Reducing Inflammation

Chronic inflammation is a key driver of many chronic diseases, including heart disease, and many spices and herbs have powerful anti-inflammatory properties. For example, turmeric, a spice commonly used in Indian and Middle Eastern cuisine, contains a compound called curcumin that has been shown to reduce inflammation in the body. Other anti-inflammatory spices and herbs include ginger, garlic, cinnamon, and rosemary.

2. Improving Cholesterol Levels

Several spices and herbs have been shown to have direct cholesterol-lowering effects. For example, fenugreek, a spice commonly used in Indian and North African cuisine, contains compounds called saponins that can help reduce total and LDL cholesterol levels. Other cholesterol-lowering spices and herbs include coriander, ginger, and black pepper.

3. Enhancing Antioxidant Activity

Many spices and herbs are rich in antioxidants, which can help protect against oxidative stress and inflammation in the body. For example, oregano, a herb commonly used in Mediterranean and Mexican cuisine, is one of the most antioxidant-rich foods on the planet, containing high levels of compounds called phenols and flavonoids. Other antioxidant-rich spices and herbs include cloves, cinnamon, and sage.

4. Supporting Healthy Blood Sugar Levels

Some spices and herbs have been shown to help regulate blood sugar levels, which can be beneficial for people with diabetes or metabolic syndrome, both of which are risk factors for heart disease. For example, cinnamon has been shown to improve insulin sensitivity and reduce fasting blood sugar levels, while fenugreek has been shown to slow the absorption of sugar in the digestive tract.

Incorporating Spices and Herbs into Your Cooking

Now that we have a better understanding of the cholesterol-lowering properties of spices and herbs, let's take a closer look at some practical ways to incorporate more of these flavorful ingredients into your daily diet.

1. Spice Up Your Breakfast

Starting your day with a spice-rich breakfast can be a great way to set the tone for a heart-healthy day. Try adding a sprinkle of cinnamon to your morning oatmeal or yogurt, or whipping up a batch of savory breakfast muffins flavored with herbs like rosemary or thyme.

2. Embrace Bold Flavors at Lunch

Lunchtime is a great opportunity to experiment with bolder, more assertive flavors from spices and herbs. Try adding a pinch of cumin or smoked paprika to your lunchtime salads, or stirring a spoonful of harissa or chimichurri into your soup or stew.

3. Make Dinner a Spice Odyssey

Dinnertime is when many people have the most time and energy to devote to cooking, so it's a great opportunity to really explore the world of spices and herbs. Try experimenting with different ethnic cuisines that are known for their bold, complex flavors, such as Indian, Thai, or Ethiopian. Or, simply start by adding a new spice or herb to one of your favorite dinner recipes each week, and see how it transforms the dish.

4. Don't Forget the Garnishes

Garnishes are not just a pretty addition to your plate; they can also be a great way to sneak in some extra heart-healthy spices and herbs. Try topping your soups and stews with a sprinkle of fresh cilantro or parsley, or adding a dollop of spice-rich chutney or salsa to your grilled meats or roasted vegetables.

5. Sip on Spice-Infused Beverages

Beverages are another great way to incorporate more spices and herbs into your diet. Try steeping a pot of chai tea with cinnamon, cardamom, and ginger, or blending up a smoothie with a pinch of cayenne pepper or turmeric for an extra anti-inflammatory boost.

DIY Spice Blends and Herb-Infused Recipes

One of the best ways to make spices and herbs a regular part of your diet is to have a few go-to blends and recipes on hand that you can whip up quickly and easily. Here are a few ideas to get you started:

1. All-Purpose Spice Blend

This versatile blend can be used to add flavor and nutrition to everything from roasted vegetables to grilled meats to soups and stews. Simply mix together equal parts cumin, coriander, paprika, and turmeric, and store in an airtight container for up to six months.

2. Herbes de Provence

This classic French blend is a great way to add a touch of Mediterranean flavor to your cooking. Mix together equal parts dried basil, thyme, oregano, and rosemary, along with a pinch of fennel seeds and lavender (if desired). Use to season roasted chicken, grilled fish, or even simple pasta dishes.

3. Curry Powder

Curry powder is a staple of Indian and Southeast Asian cuisine, and it's a great way to add a ton of flavor and nutrition to your meals. Mix together equal parts cumin, coriander, turmeric, and ginger, along with a pinch of cayenne pepper and cardamom (if desired). Use to season lentil soups, vegetable stir-fries, or even scrambled eggs.

4. Chimichurri Sauce

This zesty Argentinian sauce is packed with heart-healthy herbs and spices, including parsley, cilantro, garlic, and red pepper flakes. Simply blend together a bunch of fresh parsley and cilantro with a few cloves of garlic, a splash of red wine vinegar, and a pinch of red pepper flakes. Drizzle over grilled meats, roasted vegetables, or even use as a dip for crusty bread.

5. Golden Milk

This soothing, anti-inflammatory beverage is a great way to wind down at the end of the day. Simply heat up a cup of unsweetened almond or coconut milk with a teaspoon of turmeric, a pinch of cinnamon and ginger, and a dash of black pepper (which helps boost the absorption of curcumin). Sweeten with a touch of honey or maple syrup, if desired.

The Bottom Line on Spices and Herbs for Heart Health

Incorporating more spices and herbs into your diet is a simple, delicious way to boost your heart health and lower your cholesterol levels. These flavorful ingredients are packed with antioxidants, anti-inflammatory compounds, and other beneficial nutrients that can help protect against chronic disease and promote overall wellness.

By experimenting with different spice blends and herb-infused recipes, you can easily add more variety, flavor, and nutrition to your meals, without sacrificing taste or satisfaction. And by making these small changes a regular part of your cooking routine, you can start to reap the cumulative benefits of these powerful allies in the battle against cholesterol and heart disease.

So go ahead and spice up your life! Your heart (and your taste buds) will thank you.

CHAPTER 9

Chapter 9: Lifestyle Changes for a Healthier Heart

While diet plays a crucial role in managing cholesterol levels and promoting heart health, it's just one piece of the puzzle. To truly optimize your cardiovascular well-being, it's important to take a holistic approach that encompasses all aspects of your lifestyle, from the way you move your body to the way you manage stress and prioritize sleep.

In this chapter, we will explore the key lifestyle factors that can have a profound impact on your heart health, and provide practical tips and strategies for making small, sustainable changes that can add up to big results over time. Whether you're just starting out on your heart-health journey or looking to take your wellness to the next level, this chapter will give you the tools and inspiration you need to transform your lifestyle and reduce your risk of heart disease.

The Importance of Regular Exercise for Cholesterol Management

Exercise is one of the most powerful tools we have for managing cholesterol levels and promoting overall heart health. When you engage in regular physical activity, you're not only burning calories and improving your cardiovascular fitness, but you're also helping to:

1. Raise HDL Cholesterol Levels

HDL, or high-density lipoprotein, is often referred to as "good" cholesterol because it helps remove excess LDL (or "bad") cholesterol from the bloodstream and transport it back to the liver for processing. Regular exercise has been shown to increase HDL cholesterol levels, which can help reduce your risk of heart disease.

2. Lower LDL Cholesterol Levels

In addition to raising HDL levels, regular exercise can also help lower LDL cholesterol levels. This is because physical activity helps improve the body's ability to use insulin, which can help reduce the amount of LDL cholesterol produced by the liver.

3. Reduce Triglyceride Levels

Triglycerides are another type of fat found in the bloodstream that can contribute to the development of heart disease when levels are high. Regular exercise has been shown to help lower triglyceride levels, especially when combined with a healthy diet that's low in refined carbs and added sugars.

4. Improve Circulation

When you exercise, your heart rate increases and your blood vessels dilate, which helps improve circulation throughout the body. This can help reduce your risk of developing blood clots and other circulatory problems that can contribute to heart disease.

5. Manage Stress and Improve Mental Health

Exercise is also a powerful tool for managing stress and promoting overall mental health, both of which can have a big impact on your heart health. When you're stressed, your body releases hormones like cortisol and adrenaline that can raise your blood pressure and increase inflammation throughout the body. Regular exercise can help reduce stress levels and improve mood, which can help lower your risk of heart disease over time.

So, how much exercise do you need to reap these heart-healthy benefits? The American Heart Association recommends getting at least 150 minutes of moderate-intensity aerobic exercise (like brisk walking or cycling) or 75 minutes of vigorous-intensity aerobic exercise (like jogging or swimming) per week, along with two to three sessions of strength training exercise.

But if you're just starting out, don't feel like you need to hit these targets right away. Even small amounts of physical activity can make a big difference in your heart health over time. Start with just 10-15 minutes of exercise per day, and gradually work your way up to longer and more frequent sessions as your fitness level improves.

Stress Reduction Techniques for Better Heart Health

Stress is a major risk factor for heart disease, and for good reason. When you're stressed, your body goes into "fight or flight" mode, releasing hormones that can raise your blood pressure, increase inflammation, and put extra strain on your heart.

Over time, chronic stress can take a serious toll on your cardiovascular health, increasing your risk of heart attack, stroke, and other serious complications. That's why it's so important to prioritize stress reduction as part of your overall heart-health plan.

Here are some effective stress reduction techniques that can help lower your risk of heart disease:

1. Mindfulness Meditation

Mindfulness meditation is a simple but powerful technique that involves focusing your attention on the present moment, without judgment. By practicing mindfulness regularly, you can help reduce stress and anxiety, improve your mood, and even lower your blood pressure and heart rate.

To get started with mindfulness meditation, find a quiet, comfortable place to sit or lie down. Close your eyes and focus your attention on your breath, noticing the sensation of the air moving in and out of your body. If your mind starts to wander (which it probably will), gently redirect your attention back to your breath. Start with just a few minutes of meditation per day, and gradually work your way up to longer sessions as you become more comfortable with the practice.

2. Deep Breathing Exercises

Deep breathing is another simple but effective stress reduction technique that can help lower your heart rate and blood pressure, and promote a sense of calm and relaxation.

To practice deep breathing, find a comfortable seated position and place one hand on your chest and the other on your belly. Take a slow, deep breath in through your nose, allowing your belly to expand as you inhale. Hold the breath for a count of three, then exhale slowly through your mouth, allowing your belly to fall as you exhale. Repeat this process for several minutes, focusing your attention on the sensation of the breath moving in and out of your body.

3. Yoga and Tai Chi

Yoga and tai chi are two ancient practices that combine gentle movement, deep breathing, and mindfulness to promote stress reduction and overall well-being.

Both practices have been shown to have significant benefits for heart health, including lowering blood pressure, reducing inflammation, and improving circulation. They can also help improve flexibility, balance, and strength, which can help reduce your risk of falls and other injuries as you age.

If you're new to yoga or tai chi, consider taking a beginner's class or working with a certified instructor to learn the basic movements and techniques. As you become more comfortable with the practice, you can gradually incorporate longer and more challenging sessions into your routine.

4. Spending Time in Nature

Spending time in nature has been shown to have significant benefits for stress reduction and overall well-being. Whether you're taking a walk in the park, going for a hike in the woods, or simply sitting outside and enjoying the fresh air, being in nature can help lower your heart rate and blood pressure, reduce stress and anxiety, and promote a sense of calm and relaxation.

Try to incorporate nature time into your daily routine, even if it's just for a few minutes a day. Take a walk during your lunch break, sit outside while you enjoy your morning coffee, or plan a weekend hike with friends or family.

5. Connecting with Others

Social connection is another important factor in stress reduction and heart health. When you have strong social connections and a supportive network of friends and family, you're better able to cope with stress and maintain a positive outlook on life.

Make an effort to prioritize social connection in your daily life, whether it's through regular phone calls or video chats with loved ones, joining a club or group that shares your interests, or simply making time for coffee or dinner with friends.

By incorporating these stress reduction techniques into your daily routine, you can help lower your risk of heart disease and improve your overall well-being. Remember, stress management is a skill that takes practice and patience – so be kind to yourself as you navigate the process, and celebrate the small victories along the way.

Quitting Smoking and Limiting Alcohol Consumption

In addition to regular exercise and stress reduction, there are two other key lifestyle changes that can have a big impact on your heart health: quitting smoking and limiting alcohol consumption.

Smoking is one of the biggest risk factors for heart disease, and for good reason. The chemicals in cigarette smoke can damage the lining of your arteries, increase inflammation throughout your body, and raise your blood pressure and heart rate. Over time, this can lead to the development of plaque in your arteries, which can narrow or block blood flow to your heart and increase your risk of heart attack and stroke.

If you currently smoke, quitting is one of the best things you can do for your heart health. While quitting can be challenging, there are many resources and support systems available to help you through the process, including nicotine replacement therapy, prescription medications, and support groups.

Limiting alcohol consumption is another important step in protecting your heart health. While moderate alcohol consumption (defined as up to one drink per day for women and up to two drinks per day for men) has been associated with some potential heart health benefits, excessive alcohol consumption can have the opposite effect.

Heavy drinking can raise your blood pressure, increase inflammation throughout your body, and contribute to the development of arrhythmias (irregular heartbeats) and other heart problems. It can also interfere with the effectiveness of certain medications, including those used to treat high blood pressure and high cholesterol.

If you choose to drink alcohol, it's important to do so in moderation and to be mindful of the potential risks. If you're concerned about your alcohol consumption or have a history of alcohol abuse, talk to your doctor or a mental health professional about strategies for cutting back or quitting altogether.

Making Lifestyle Changes for a Healthier Heart: Where to Start

Making lifestyle changes can be challenging, especially if you've been living a certain way for a long time. But the good news is that even small changes can make a big difference in your heart health over time.

If you're not sure where to start, here are some simple steps you can take to begin incorporating heart-healthy habits into your daily routine:

1. Set realistic goals. Instead of trying to overhaul your entire lifestyle overnight, focus on making small, achievable changes that you can sustain over time. For example, if you're not currently exercising regularly, start by committing to a 10-minute walk each day and gradually work your way up to longer and more frequent sessions.

2. Find activities you enjoy. Exercise doesn't have to be a chore – in fact, it's much easier to stick with an exercise routine if you actually enjoy the activities you're doing. Experiment with different types of exercise, like dancing, hiking, or swimming, until you find something that feels fun and rewarding.

3. Make time for stress reduction. Stress management is just as important as exercise when it comes to heart health, so make sure to carve out time each day for activities that help you feel calm and centered. Whether it's a few minutes of deep breathing, a yoga class, or a conversation with a trusted friend, prioritizing stress reduction can have a big impact on your overall well-being.

4. Plan ahead. One of the biggest barriers to making healthy lifestyle changes is lack of time and energy. To make things easier on yourself, try planning ahead as much as possible. Prep healthy meals and snacks in advance, lay out your workout clothes the night before, and schedule your stress reduction activities like you would any other important appointment.

5. Celebrate your successes. Making lifestyle changes can be challenging, so it's important to celebrate your successes along the way. Whether it's hitting a new personal best in your workout routine or going a whole week without smoking, take time to acknowledge and appreciate the progress you're making.

Remember, making lifestyle changes for a healthier heart is a journey, not a destination. There will be ups and downs along the way, but by staying committed to your goals and being kind to yourself in the process, you can create lasting, positive changes that will benefit your health and well-being for years to come.

CHAPTER 10

Chapter 10: Supplements for Cholesterol Support: Separating Fact from Fiction

In the world of natural health and wellness, supplements have long been touted as a simple and effective way to support various aspects of health, including cholesterol management. From omega-3 fatty acids to fiber and beyond, there's no shortage of supplements claiming to help lower cholesterol levels and promote heart health.

But with so many options available, it can be challenging to separate fact from fiction and determine which supplements, if any, are worth incorporating into your cholesterol management plan. In this chapter, we'll take a closer look at some of the most popular cholesterol-lowering supplements on the market, exploring the science behind their claims and weighing the potential benefits and risks of each.

Whether you're considering adding a new supplement to your routine or simply curious about the latest trends in natural cholesterol management, this chapter will provide you with the information and insights you need to make informed decisions about your health.

Evaluating the Effectiveness of Popular Cholesterol-Lowering Supplements
Before we dive into specific supplements, it's important to understand how we evaluate the effectiveness of these products. When it comes to supplements

for cholesterol management, there are a few key factors to consider:

1. Scientific evidence: Is there solid scientific research to support the claims made about the supplement? Have studies been conducted in humans, and if so, what were the results?

2. Safety: Are there any known side effects or risks associated with the supplement? Are there any potential interactions with medications or other supplements?

3. Quality: Is the supplement manufactured by a reputable company with strict quality control standards? Has it been third-party tested for purity and potency?

4. Cost: Is the supplement affordable and accessible, or is it prohibitively expensive?

With these factors in mind, let's take a closer look at some of the most popular cholesterol-lowering supplements on the market today.

Omega-3 Fatty Acids

Omega-3 fatty acids, found naturally in fatty fish and fish oil supplements, have long been touted for their heart-healthy benefits. These essential fatty acids have been shown to help reduce inflammation, lower triglyceride levels, and improve HDL (good) cholesterol levels in some studies.

However, the evidence for omega-3s as a cholesterol-lowering supplement is mixed. While some studies have shown modest reductions in LDL (bad) cholesterol levels with fish oil supplementation, others have found no significant effect. Additionally, high doses of omega-3 supplements can cause side effects like digestive upset and increased bleeding risk in some people.

If you're considering taking an omega-3 supplement for cholesterol management, it's important to talk to your doctor first. They can help you weigh the potential benefits and risks based on your individual health status and medication regimen.

Soluble Fiber

Soluble fiber, found naturally in foods like oats, barley, and legumes, has been shown to help lower LDL cholesterol levels by binding to bile acids in the digestive tract and preventing their reabsorption. This process can also help reduce the amount of cholesterol produced by the liver.

While it's always best to get your fiber from whole food sources, fiber supplements can be a convenient way to boost your intake if you're struggling to meet your daily needs through diet alone. Psyllium husk, a type of soluble fiber derived from the seeds of the Plantago ovata plant, is a popular choice for cholesterol management.

Studies have shown that taking psyllium husk supplements can help lower LDL cholesterol levels by an average of 5-10% when taken consistently over several weeks or months. However, it's important to start with a low dose and gradually increase over time to minimize digestive side effects like bloating and gas.

If you're considering taking a fiber supplement for cholesterol management, be sure to choose a high-quality product from a reputable brand, and always follow the dosing instructions carefully. It's also important to drink plenty of water when taking fiber supplements to prevent constipation and other digestive issues.

Red Yeast Rice

Red yeast rice is a traditional Chinese medicine that's gained popularity in recent years as a natural alternative to statin drugs for cholesterol management. This supplement is derived from a type of yeast that grows on rice and contains compounds called monacolins, which are structurally similar to the active ingredients in statin medications.

Studies have shown that taking red yeast rice supplements can help lower LDL cholesterol levels by an average of 20-30% when taken consistently over several weeks or months. However, the effectiveness of red yeast rice supplements can vary widely depending on the specific product and manufacturing process used.

Additionally, red yeast rice supplements can cause many of the same side effects as statin drugs, including muscle pain and liver damage in rare cases. They can also interact with certain medications, including blood thinners and calcium channel blockers.

If you're considering taking a red yeast rice supplement for cholesterol management, it's crucial to talk to your doctor first. They can help you determine whether this supplement is safe and appropriate for you based on your individual health status and medication regimen.

Garlic

Garlic has been used for centuries as a natural remedy for a variety of health conditions, including high cholesterol. This pungent herb contains compounds called allicin and S-allyl cysteine, which have been shown to have cholesterol-lowering properties in some studies.

While the evidence for garlic as a cholesterol-lowering supplement is mixed, some studies have shown modest reductions in total and LDL cholesterol levels with garlic supplementation. However, the effectiveness of garlic supplements can vary widely depending on the specific product and dosage used.

Additionally, garlic supplements can cause side effects like bad breath, body odor, and digestive upset in some people. They can also interact with certain medications, including blood thinners and HIV medications.

If you're considering taking a garlic supplement for cholesterol management, it's important to choose a high-quality product from a reputable brand and follow the dosing instructions carefully. You should also talk to your doctor first to ensure that garlic supplementation is safe and appropriate for you.

Plant Sterols and Stanols

Plant sterols and stanols are naturally occurring compounds found in small amounts in many plant-based foods, including vegetables, fruits, nuts, and seeds. These compounds have a similar structure to cholesterol and can help block its absorption in the digestive tract.

Studies have shown that consuming 2-3 grams of plant sterols or stanols per day can help lower LDL cholesterol levels by an average of 10-15% when consumed consistently over several weeks or months. However, it can be challenging to get this amount through diet alone, which is where supplements come in.

Plant sterol and stanol supplements are widely available in the form of capsules, tablets, and fortified foods like margarine and orange juice. These supplements are generally considered safe and well-tolerated, with few reported side effects.

However, it's important to note that plant sterols and stanols can interfere with the absorption of certain fat-soluble vitamins, including vitamins A, D, E, and K. If you're taking a plant sterol or stanol supplement, it's a good idea to ensure that you're getting enough of these vitamins through diet or additional supplementation.

If you're considering taking a plant sterol or stanol supplement for cholesterol management, be sure to choose a high-quality product from a reputable brand and follow the dosing instructions carefully. As with any supplement, it's always a good idea to talk to your doctor first to ensure that it's safe and appropriate for you.

Potential Risks and Interactions of Supplements

While supplements can be a useful tool for cholesterol management in some cases, it's important to remember that they are not without risks. Even natural supplements can cause side effects and interact with medications, so it's crucial to approach them with caution and care.

Some potential risks and interactions to be aware of when taking cholesterol-lowering supplements include:

1. Digestive upset: Supplements like fiber and garlic can cause bloating, gas, and other digestive issues in some people, particularly when taken in high doses or on an empty stomach.

2. Nutrient interactions: Some supplements, like plant sterols and stanols, can interfere with the absorption of certain nutrients when taken in high doses or over an extended period.

3. Medication interactions: Many supplements can interact with prescription medications, either reducing their effectiveness or increasing the risk of side effects. It's crucial to talk to your doctor about any supplements you're considering taking if you're on medication.

4. Quality concerns: The supplement industry is largely unregulated, which means that the quality and purity of supplements can vary widely from brand to brand. It's important to choose supplements from reputable companies that follow strict quality control standards and have their products third-party tested for purity and potency.

Ultimately, the decision to take a cholesterol-lowering supplement should be made in consultation with your healthcare provider, taking into account your individual health status, medication regimen, and overall goals for cholesterol management.

When to Consider Supplements Under Medical Supervision

While lifestyle changes like diet and exercise should always be the first line of defense against high cholesterol, there may be cases where supplements can be a useful addition to your cholesterol management plan. However, it's important to approach supplements with caution and always use them under the guidance of a qualified healthcare professional.

Some situations where your doctor may recommend a cholesterol-lowering supplement include:

1. If you have significantly elevated LDL cholesterol levels that are not responding to lifestyle changes alone
2. If you have a genetic condition that makes it difficult to manage cholesterol levels through diet and exercise alone
3. If you are unable to tolerate statin medications due to side effects or other medical conditions
4. If you have a documented nutrient deficiency that is contributing to high cholesterol levels

In these cases, your doctor may recommend a specific supplement or combination of supplements based on your individual needs and health status. They will also monitor your response to the supplement over time, adjusting the dosage or discontinuing use as needed based on your cholesterol levels and overall health.

It's important to remember that supplements should never be used as a substitute for a healthy lifestyle or prescribed medications. While they can be a useful tool in some cases, they are not a magic bullet for cholesterol management and should always be used in conjunction with other evidence-based strategies for heart health.

Conclusion

When it comes to supplements for cholesterol management, the world of natural health and wellness can be a confusing and overwhelming place. With so many products and claims to navigate, it can be challenging to separate fact from fiction and determine which supplements, if any, are worth incorporating into your cholesterol management plan.

However, by approaching supplements with a critical eye and a commitment to evidence-based health practices, it is possible to make informed decisions about your cholesterol management strategy. Whether you're considering omega-3 fatty acids, soluble fiber, red yeast rice, garlic, or plant sterols and stanols, it's crucial to do your research, consult with your healthcare provider, and choose high-quality products from reputable brands.

Ultimately, while supplements can be a useful tool in some cases, they should never be used as a substitute for a healthy lifestyle or prescribed medications. The foundation of any effective cholesterol management plan should always be a nutrient-rich diet, regular exercise, stress management, and other lifestyle factors that promote overall heart health.

By prioritizing these foundational strategies and using supplements judiciously under medical supervision, you can take a proactive and personalized approach to cholesterol management that supports your long-term health and well-being. So don't be afraid to ask questions, do your research, and work closely with your healthcare team to develop a cholesterol management plan that works for you. Your heart will thank you for it!

CHAPTER 11

Chapter 11: Partnering with Your Healthcare Provider

When it comes to managing your cholesterol levels and overall heart health, working closely with your healthcare provider is essential. Your doctor can provide personalized guidance and support based on your unique health history, risk factors, and goals, helping you navigate the often-complex world of cholesterol management with confidence and clarity.

In this chapter, we'll explore the importance of regular check-ups and cholesterol screenings, discuss strategies for communicating effectively with your healthcare team, and provide guidance on when medication may be necessary alongside lifestyle changes. By partnering with your healthcare provider and taking an active role in your own health journey, you can optimize your cholesterol management plan and set yourself up for long-term success.

The Importance of Regular Check-Ups and Cholesterol Screenings

One of the most important things you can do for your cholesterol and overall heart health is to stay up-to-date with regular check-ups and screenings. These routine visits provide an opportunity for your healthcare provider to assess your current health status, monitor any changes over time, and provide personalized recommendations for managing your cholesterol levels.

During a typical check-up, your doctor will likely perform a physical exam, measure your blood pressure and weight, and ask about any symptoms or concerns you may have. They may also order blood tests to check your cholesterol levels, as well as other important markers of heart health like blood sugar, triglycerides, and inflammation.

The frequency of these check-ups and screenings may vary depending on your age, health status, and risk factors for heart disease. However, the American Heart Association generally recommends that all adults have their cholesterol levels checked at least once every 4-6 years, starting at age 20. If you have a family history of heart disease, high cholesterol, or other risk factors, your doctor may recommend more frequent screenings.

It's important to keep in mind that high cholesterol often has no symptoms, which means that regular screenings are the only way to know if your levels are in a healthy range. By staying on top of these check-ups and screenings, you can catch any potential issues early on and work with your healthcare provider to develop a plan for managing your cholesterol and reducing your risk of heart disease.

Discussing Your Cholesterol-Lowering Plan with Your Doctor

If your cholesterol levels are found to be high during a routine screening, the next step is to work with your healthcare provider to develop a personalized plan for managing them. This plan may include a combination of lifestyle changes, such as diet and exercise modifications, as well as medication if necessary.

When discussing your cholesterol management plan with your doctor, it's important to be open and honest about your current lifestyle habits, any challenges or barriers you may face in making changes, and your overall goals for heart health. Some key topics to cover may include:

1. Your current diet and exercise habits: Be honest about what you typically

eat and how much physical activity you get on a regular basis. This information can help your doctor provide more targeted recommendations for making heart-healthy changes.

2. Your family history of heart disease: If you have a family history of high cholesterol, heart attack, or stroke, be sure to share this information with your doctor. This can help them assess your individual risk factors and recommend appropriate screening and management strategies.

3. Any medications or supplements you are currently taking: It's important to provide your doctor with a complete list of all the medications and supplements you are taking, including over-the-counter products and herbal remedies. Some of these products may interact with cholesterol-lowering medications or affect your overall heart health.

4. Your personal preferences and goals: Be clear about your preferences for managing your cholesterol, whether that means focusing on lifestyle changes, considering medication, or a combination of both. It's also important to discuss your overall goals for heart health and any concerns or questions you may have about the management process.

By having an open and honest conversation with your healthcare provider about your cholesterol management plan, you can work together to develop a strategy that is tailored to your individual needs and preferences. This collaborative approach can help you feel more empowered and motivated to make lasting changes for better heart health.

When Medication May Be Necessary Alongside Lifestyle Changes

While lifestyle changes like diet and exercise are often the first line of defense against high cholesterol, there may be cases where medication is necessary to help lower levels and reduce the risk of heart disease. The decision to start medication for cholesterol management is one that should be made in close consultation with your healthcare provider, taking into account your individual health status, risk factors, and overall goals.

Some situations where your doctor may recommend cholesterol-lowering medication include:

1. If your LDL cholesterol levels are very high (190 mg/dL or above) and lifestyle changes alone are not enough to lower them sufficiently
2. If you have a history of heart attack, stroke, or other cardiovascular events, even if your cholesterol levels are not severely elevated
3. If you have diabetes, which increases your risk of heart disease and may require more aggressive cholesterol management
4. If you have a family history of early heart disease (before age 55 in men or before age 65 in women), which may indicate a genetic predisposition to high cholesterol

The most common type of medication used to lower cholesterol is a class of drugs called statins. Statins work by blocking an enzyme in the liver that is involved in the production of cholesterol, helping to reduce the amount of LDL cholesterol in the bloodstream. Some common examples of statin medications include atorvastatin (Lipitor), rosuvastatin (Crestor), and simvastatin (Zocor).

While statins are generally considered safe and effective for most people, they can cause side effects in some cases. These may include muscle pain or weakness, digestive issues, or liver damage in rare cases. If you experience any concerning symptoms while taking a statin medication, it's important to let your doctor know right away so that they can adjust your treatment plan as needed.

In addition to statins, there are several other types of cholesterol-lowering medications that may be recommended in certain cases. These include:

1. Bile acid sequestrants: These drugs work by binding to bile acids in the digestive tract, which helps to remove cholesterol from the body. Examples include cholestyramine (Questran) and colesevelam (Welchol).

2. Cholesterol absorption inhibitors: These drugs work by blocking the absorption of cholesterol in the intestines, helping to lower LDL levels. The most common example is ezetimibe (Zetia).

3. PCSK9 inhibitors: These newer drugs work by blocking a protein that interferes with the liver's ability to remove LDL cholesterol from the bloodstream. Examples include alirocumab (Praluent) and evolocumab (Repatha).

It's important to keep in mind that while medication can be an effective tool for managing high cholesterol, it should always be used in combination with lifestyle changes for optimal results. In some cases, making significant changes to your diet and exercise habits may allow you to reduce or even eliminate the need for medication over time, with guidance from your healthcare provider.

Monitoring Your Progress and Adjusting Your Plan as Needed

Once you have developed a cholesterol management plan with your healthcare provider, it's important to monitor your progress over time and make adjustments as needed based on your individual response and evolving health needs.

Your doctor will likely recommend regular follow-up visits and blood tests to track your cholesterol levels and assess the effectiveness of your current management strategies. These visits provide an opportunity to discuss any challenges or concerns you may have, celebrate your successes, and make any necessary adjustments to your plan.

Some key markers of progress to track over time may include:

1. LDL cholesterol levels: The primary goal of cholesterol management is to lower LDL (bad) cholesterol levels to a healthy range, typically below 100 mg/dL for most people. Your doctor will monitor your LDL levels regularly to ensure that your current plan is working effectively.

2. HDL cholesterol levels: While the focus of cholesterol management is often on lowering LDL levels, it's also important to maintain healthy levels of HDL (good) cholesterol. In general, an HDL level of 60 mg/dL or higher is considered protective against heart disease.

3. Triglyceride levels: High triglyceride levels can also contribute to heart disease risk, so your doctor may monitor these levels along with your cholesterol. A healthy triglyceride level is typically below 150 mg/dL.

4. Other markers of heart health: Depending on your individual health status and risk factors, your doctor may also monitor other markers of heart health, such as blood pressure, blood sugar, and inflammation levels.

If your cholesterol levels are not improving as expected or you are experiencing side effects from medication, your doctor may recommend adjusting your treatment plan. This may involve changing the dose or type of medication you are taking, modifying your diet and exercise habits, or exploring other lifestyle factors that may be contributing to your cholesterol levels.

It's important to be patient and persistent in your cholesterol management efforts, as it can take time to see significant changes in your levels. However, by working closely with your healthcare provider and staying committed to your plan, you can make steady progress towards better heart health over time.

The Bottom Line on Partnering with Your Healthcare Provider

Managing your cholesterol levels and overall heart health is a team effort, and your healthcare provider is a key player on that team. By staying up-to-date with regular check-ups and screenings, communicating openly and honestly about your goals and challenges, and working collaboratively to develop and adjust your management plan over time, you can optimize your cholesterol levels and reduce your risk of heart disease.

It's important to remember that while your healthcare provider can provide guidance and support, ultimately the day-to-day choices that impact your heart health are up to you. By taking an active role in your own health journey, staying informed about your options, and being proactive about making positive changes, you can become your own best advocate for better cholesterol management and overall wellness.

So don't hesitate to partner with your healthcare provider and take charge of your cholesterol health today. With the right combination of medical guidance, lifestyle changes, and personalized support, you can achieve your goals and enjoy a healthier, more vibrant life for years to come.

CHAPTER 12

Chapter 12: Success Stories: Real People, Real Results

Throughout this book, we've explored the many ways in which individuals can lower their cholesterol levels naturally, from adopting a heart-healthy diet and exercise routine to incorporating targeted supplements and partnering with healthcare providers. But what does this journey look like in practice, and what kind of results can people realistically expect to achieve?

In this chapter, we'll take a closer look at the stories of real individuals who have successfully lowered their cholesterol levels through natural means. These inspiring stories showcase the power of lifestyle changes and personalized strategies in transforming cardiovascular health, and offer valuable lessons and insights for anyone looking to embark on their own cholesterol-lowering journey.

From small, sustainable shifts to major overhauls in diet and lifestyle, these success stories demonstrate the many different paths to better heart health, and the incredible resilience and determination of those who have taken control of their cholesterol levels and overall well-being. So let's dive in and explore the triumphs, challenges, and transformative experiences of these everyday heroes.

Sarah's Story: A Wakeup Call and a New Way of Eating

Sarah, a 45-year-old mother of two, had always considered herself relatively healthy, despite carrying a few extra pounds and leading a busy, stressful life. However, a routine check-up with her doctor revealed that her cholesterol levels were alarmingly high, with an LDL level of 190 mg/dL and an HDL level of just 35 mg/dL.

Shocked and scared by these results, Sarah knew she needed to make some changes, but she wasn't sure where to start. Her doctor recommended a statin medication, but Sarah was hesitant to rely solely on drugs to manage her cholesterol. Instead, she decided to explore natural options first, starting with a complete overhaul of her diet.

With the help of a registered dietitian, Sarah learned about the power of a plant-based, whole-foods diet in lowering cholesterol levels naturally. She gradually transitioned away from processed, high-fat foods and incorporated more fruits, vegetables, whole grains, legumes, and healthy plant-based fats into her meals.

At first, the changes felt overwhelming, and Sarah struggled with cravings for her old favorite foods. But as she experimented with new recipes and discovered delicious, satisfying plant-based meals, she began to enjoy the process of nourishing her body with wholesome, nutrient-dense foods.

Over time, Sarah's hard work and dedication paid off. After just three months of following her new diet plan, her LDL cholesterol had dropped to 130 mg/dL, and her HDL had increased to 45 mg/dL. Encouraged by these results, Sarah continued to refine and expand her healthy eating habits, incorporating more variety and flavor into her meals while staying true to her plant-based principles.

Today, two years after her initial wake-up call, Sarah's cholesterol levels are well within the healthy range, with an LDL of 95 mg/dL and an HDL of 60 mg/dL. But the benefits of her lifestyle changes go far beyond the numbers.

Sarah reports feeling more energetic, clear-headed, and confident in her ability to make positive choices for her health and well-being. She has even inspired her family to adopt healthier habits, creating a ripple effect of positive change in her community.

Sarah's story is a powerful reminder that even small, gradual changes in diet can have a profound impact on cholesterol levels and overall health. By focusing on whole, plant-based foods and staying committed to her goals, Sarah was able to transform her cardiovascular health and reclaim her vitality, one meal at a time.

John's Journey: Fitness, Function, and a New Lease on Life

John, a 60-year-old retired accountant, had always been relatively active, enjoying daily walks and the occasional round of golf. However, a diagnosis of high cholesterol and borderline diabetes served as a wake-up call, forcing John to reassess his lifestyle and make some changes to protect his heart health.

With a starting LDL cholesterol level of 160 mg/dL and an HDL level of 40 mg/dL, John knew he needed to take action. His doctor prescribed a statin medication, but John was determined to explore natural options as well. He had heard about the benefits of exercise in lowering cholesterol and improving overall cardiovascular function, and he decided to make physical activity a top priority in his cholesterol management plan.

John started slowly, gradually increasing the duration and intensity of his daily walks. He also joined a local fitness center and began working with a personal trainer to develop a safe, effective exercise routine that included a mix of cardio and strength training. At first, the workouts were challenging, and John sometimes felt discouraged by his limitations. But as he continued to show up and put in the effort, he began to notice improvements in his stamina, strength, and overall sense of well-being.

As John's fitness level improved, he began to explore new activities and challenges. He joined a hiking group and discovered a love for outdoor adventure, setting goals to conquer local trails and even take on a multi-day backpacking trip. He also started playing tennis with friends, enjoying the social connection and competitive spirit of the game.

After six months of consistent exercise and a healthy diet, John's cholesterol levels had improved significantly, with an LDL of 120 mg/dL and an HDL of 55 mg/dL. His doctor was thrilled with his progress and encouraged him to continue with his active lifestyle, noting the many benefits of exercise for cardiovascular health, weight management, and overall well-being.

Today, John is a vocal advocate for the power of physical activity in managing cholesterol and preventing chronic disease. He continues to set new fitness goals and explore new activities, and he even volunteers with a local senior center to help other older adults discover the joys and benefits of an active lifestyle.

John's journey is a testament to the transformative power of exercise in improving cholesterol levels and overall health. By starting small, staying consistent, and finding activities that he enjoyed, John was able to make physical activity a sustainable, rewarding part of his daily life, with benefits that extend far beyond the numbers on his cholesterol chart.

Maria's Mission: A Holistic Approach to Heart Health

Maria, a 50-year-old small business owner, had always been mindful of her health, but a family history of heart disease and a personal battle with stress and anxiety left her feeling vulnerable and unsure of her cardiovascular future. When a routine blood test revealed elevated cholesterol levels, with an LDL of 150 mg/dL and an HDL of 45 mg/dL, Maria knew it was time to take a proactive, holistic approach to managing her heart health.

Working closely with her healthcare provider, Maria developed a comprehensive plan that included a mix of lifestyle changes and targeted supplements. She began by focusing on her diet, incorporating more cholesterol-lowering foods like fruits, vegetables, whole grains, and lean proteins. She also experimented with stress-reducing practices like meditation, yoga, and deep breathing, finding that these techniques helped her feel more centered and resilient in the face of daily challenges.

In addition to these lifestyle changes, Maria's doctor recommended a few key supplements to support her cholesterol management efforts. These included omega-3 fatty acids to help lower triglycerides and reduce inflammation, plant sterols to block cholesterol absorption, and CoQ10 to support healthy heart function. Maria was initially hesitant about adding supplements to her regimen, but with careful research and guidance from her healthcare team, she found a combination that worked well for her unique needs and goals.

As Maria continued to implement her holistic heart health plan, she began to notice improvements in her energy levels, mood, and overall sense of well-being. Her cholesterol levels also began to improve, with her LDL dropping to 130 mg/dL and her HDL increasing to 55 mg/dL after just three months of consistent effort.

Encouraged by these results, Maria continued to refine and expand her approach, incorporating new stress-reducing practices and experimenting with different cholesterol-lowering foods and supplements. She also began to share her journey with others, using her business platform to raise awareness about the importance of holistic heart health and inspire her employees and customers to prioritize their own well-being.

Today, Maria's cholesterol levels are well within the healthy range, and she continues to embrace a holistic approach to heart health that nourishes her body, mind, and spirit. Her story is a powerful reminder that there is no one-size-fits-all approach to managing cholesterol and preventing heart disease, and that the most effective strategies are often those that address the whole person, not just the numbers on a lab report.

Lessons Learned and Tips for Staying Motivated

The success stories of Sarah, John, and Maria offer valuable insights and inspiration for anyone looking to lower their cholesterol levels naturally and reclaim their cardiovascular health. While each of their journeys was unique, there are some common themes and lessons that can help guide and motivate others on their own paths to better heart health.

1. Start small and build gradually. Whether you're overhauling your diet, starting an exercise routine, or incorporating new supplements and stress-reducing practices, it's important to start small and build gradually over time. This approach can help you avoid overwhelm, build confidence, and create sustainable habits that stick.

2. Find what works for you. There is no one-size-fits-all approach to managing cholesterol and improving heart health. What works for one person may not work for another, so it's important to experiment with different strategies and find what resonates with your unique needs, preferences, and lifestyle. Don't be afraid to try new things and adjust your plan as needed.

3. Celebrate your successes. Managing cholesterol and improving heart health is a journey, not a destination. It's important to celebrate your successes along the way, no matter how small they may seem. Whether it's a drop in your LDL levels, a new personal best in your exercise routine, or a week of consistent healthy eating, take time to acknowledge and appreciate your progress.

4. Surround yourself with support. Lowering cholesterol naturally can be a challenging and sometimes isolating process, but it's important to remember that you don't have to go it alone. Surround yourself with supportive friends, family members, and healthcare providers who can offer encouragement, guidance, and accountability on your journey.

5. Focus on the big picture. While lowering cholesterol is an important goal, it's not the only measure of success when it comes to heart health. Focus on the big picture of overall well-being, including factors like energy levels, mood, stress management, and quality of life. By taking a holistic approach and prioritizing your overall health and happiness, you can create a more resilient, fulfilling path to better cardiovascular health.

The success stories in this chapter are just a few examples of the many ways in which individuals can lower their cholesterol levels naturally and transform their cardiovascular health. By starting small, finding what works for you, celebrating your successes, surrounding yourself with support, and focusing on the big picture, you too can become a success story and inspire others on their own journeys to better heart health.

CHAPTER 13

C hapter 13: Maintaining Healthy Cholesterol Levels for Life

Congratulations! If you've made it to this chapter, you've likely experienced the transformative power of natural cholesterol management firsthand. Whether you've overhauled your diet, started a new exercise routine, incorporated targeted supplements, or all of the above, you've taken important steps towards improving your cardiovascular health and reducing your risk of heart disease.

But as with any health journey, the work doesn't stop once you've reached your initial goals. Maintaining healthy cholesterol levels for life requires ongoing effort, commitment, and resilience in the face of challenges and setbacks. In this chapter, we'll explore strategies for long-term success, navigating obstacles and staying on track, and cultivating a mindset of self-compassion and resilience as you continue on your path to optimal heart health.

Strategies for Long-Term Success

When it comes to maintaining healthy cholesterol levels for life, consistency is key. The habits and practices that helped you lower your cholesterol initially are the same ones that will help you sustain your progress over time. Here are some strategies for long-term success:

1. Make it a lifestyle, not a diet. Rather than thinking of your cholesterol-

lowering efforts as a temporary fix or a restrictive diet, try to reframe them as a lifestyle change. Focus on incorporating foods, activities, and habits that nourish your body and bring you joy, rather than feeling deprived or punished. By making healthy choices a natural, enjoyable part of your daily life, you'll be more likely to stick with them for the long haul.

2. Plan ahead and prioritize convenience. One of the biggest obstacles to maintaining healthy habits is lack of time and energy. To set yourself up for success, try to plan ahead as much as possible. Prep healthy meals and snacks in advance, schedule your exercise and self-care activities like you would any other important appointment, and keep healthy options on hand for when you're short on time or motivation.

3. Stay accountable and connected. Accountability and social support can be powerful motivators when it comes to maintaining healthy habits. Consider enlisting a friend or family member to join you on your health journey, or connect with a virtual community of like-minded individuals for encouragement and inspiration. You might also consider working with a healthcare provider or health coach who can help you set goals, track progress, and troubleshoot challenges along the way.

4. Mix things up and keep it interesting. Boredom and monotony can be major roadblocks to long-term success. To keep things fresh and engaging, try to mix up your routine from time to time. Experiment with new healthy recipes, try a different type of exercise, or explore a new stress-reducing practice. By keeping things varied and interesting, you'll be more likely to stay motivated and engaged over the long term.

5. Celebrate your successes and learn from your setbacks. Maintaining healthy cholesterol levels is a journey, not a destination. Along the way, there will be successes to celebrate and setbacks to learn from. Take time to acknowledge and appreciate your progress, no matter how small, and try to approach setbacks with curiosity and self-compassion rather than shame

or self-judgment. By viewing challenges as opportunities for growth and learning, you'll be better equipped to navigate the ups and downs of long-term cholesterol management.

Overcoming Obstacles and Staying on Track

Even with the best intentions and strategies in place, maintaining healthy cholesterol levels for life is not always a smooth or linear process. There will be times when life gets in the way, motivation wanes, or old habits creep back in. Here are some common obstacles and strategies for staying on track:

1. Travel and social events. When you're away from home or in social situations, it can be challenging to stick to your usual healthy habits. To navigate these situations, try to plan ahead as much as possible. Pack healthy snacks and meals for travel, scope out healthy options at restaurants or events, and don't be afraid to communicate your needs and preferences to others. Remember that one indulgent meal or day off track won't derail your progress, as long as you get back on track as soon as possible.

2. Stress and emotional eating. Stress and emotional triggers can be major drivers of unhealthy eating and lifestyle habits. To manage these challenges, try to develop a toolbox of healthy coping strategies, such as deep breathing, meditation, or calling a supportive friend. When you feel the urge to eat for emotional reasons, try to pause and check in with yourself. Ask yourself if you're truly hungry, or if there's another need that could be met in a healthier way.

3. Plateaus and setbacks. It's normal to experience plateaus or setbacks along the way, even if you're doing everything "right." When this happens, try not to get discouraged or give up. Instead, view these challenges as opportunities to reassess your approach and make adjustments as needed. Maybe you need to switch up your exercise routine, try a new meal planning strategy, or explore a different stress-reducing practice. Remember that setbacks are a normal part of the process, and that each one offers a chance to learn and grow.

4. Negative self-talk and perfectionism. One of the biggest obstacles to long-term success is our own inner critic. Negative self-talk and perfectionism can lead to feelings of shame, guilt, and discouragement, making it harder to stick with healthy habits over time. To combat these tendencies, try to practice self-compassion and reframe your thoughts in a more positive, supportive way. Celebrate your successes, no matter how small, and remind yourself that progress is more important than perfection.

By anticipating and preparing for these common obstacles, you'll be better equipped to stay on track and maintain your healthy cholesterol levels for the long haul. Remember that setbacks and challenges are a normal part of the journey, and that each one offers an opportunity for growth and learning.

The Importance of Self-Compassion and Resilience

As you navigate the ups and downs of maintaining healthy cholesterol levels for life, one of the most important skills you can cultivate is self-compassion. Self-compassion involves treating yourself with the same kindness, understanding, and support that you would offer to a good friend. It means acknowledging that setbacks and imperfections are a normal part of the human experience, and that your worth and value are not contingent on your ability to maintain perfect health habits all the time.

Research has shown that self-compassion is associated with a wide range of health benefits, including better mental health, greater resilience in the face of stress and adversity, and more sustainable behavior change over time. When we approach our health journey with self-compassion, we're more likely to bounce back from setbacks, stay motivated in the face of challenges, and maintain a positive, growth-oriented mindset.

So how can you cultivate self-compassion on your cholesterol management journey? Here are a few tips:

1. Practice self-kindness. When you experience a setback or challenge, try to

speak to yourself with the same kindness and understanding that you would offer to a good friend. Use supportive, encouraging language, and remind yourself that everyone makes mistakes and experiences ups and downs.

2. Embrace imperfection. Let go of the idea that you need to be perfect in order to be successful. Embrace the fact that imperfection is a normal part of the human experience, and that setbacks and challenges are opportunities for growth and learning.

3. Focus on progress, not perfection. Instead of getting caught up in the idea of achieving perfect health habits all the time, focus on making progress and taking small, consistent steps towards your goals. Celebrate your successes, no matter how small, and use setbacks as opportunities to reassess and adjust your approach.

4. Seek support and connection. Self-compassion doesn't mean going it alone. Seek out supportive friends, family members, or healthcare providers who can offer encouragement, guidance, and accountability on your journey. Remember that everyone struggles sometimes, and that asking for help is a sign of strength, not weakness.

By cultivating self-compassion and resilience on your cholesterol management journey, you'll be better equipped to navigate the ups and downs of maintaining healthy habits for life. You'll be more likely to stay motivated, bounce back from setbacks, and approach challenges with a positive, growth-oriented mindset.

Conclusion

Maintaining healthy cholesterol levels for life is a journey, not a destination. It requires ongoing effort, commitment, and resilience in the face of challenges and setbacks. But with the right strategies, mindset, and support, it is possible to sustain the benefits of natural cholesterol management over the long term.

By making healthy choices a natural, enjoyable part of your daily life, planning ahead and prioritizing convenience, staying accountable and connected, mixing things up and keeping it interesting, and celebrating your successes while learning from your setbacks, you can set yourself up for long-term success. And by cultivating self-compassion and resilience along the way, you can navigate the ups and downs of the journey with greater ease and grace.

Remember that maintaining healthy cholesterol levels is just one aspect of overall cardiovascular health and well-being. By taking a holistic approach that nourishes your body, mind, and spirit, you can create a more vibrant, fulfilling life that supports your health goals and brings you joy.

So keep going, even when the path feels challenging or uncertain. Surround yourself with support and inspiration, and trust in your own resilience and capacity for growth. With each small step and each day of consistent effort, you are building a foundation of health and well-being that will serve you for a lifetime.

CHAPTER 14

hapter 14: Recipes for a Heart-Healthy Life

Throughout this book, we've explored the many ways in which a nutritious, balanced diet can support healthy cholesterol levels and overall cardiovascular well-being. We've delved into the science behind heart-healthy eating patterns, the specific foods and nutrients that can help lower cholesterol naturally, and the strategies for making sustainable, enjoyable changes to your daily meals and snacks.

But what does this look like in practice? How can you translate the principles of heart-healthy eating into delicious, satisfying meals that nourish your body and delight your taste buds? In this final chapter, we'll bring all of these concepts together with a collection of easy-to-prepare, cholesterol-lowering recipes that showcase the best of what a heart-healthy diet has to offer.

From hearty breakfasts and lunches to flavorful dinners, snacks, and desserts, these recipes are designed to help you put your newfound knowledge into action and enjoy the many benefits of a whole-foods, plant-forward eating pattern. Each recipe includes detailed nutritional information and tips for optimizing its heart-healthy potential, so you can feel confident that you're fueling your body with the nutrients it needs to thrive.

So let's head to the kitchen and start cooking up a delicious, vibrant, heart-healthy life!

Breakfasts
1. Overnight Oats with Berries and Nuts
Ingredients:
- 1/2 cup rolled oats
- 1/2 cup unsweetened almond milk
- 1/4 cup plain Greek yogurt
- 1 tablespoon chia seeds
- 1/2 teaspoon vanilla extract
- 1/2 cup mixed berries (fresh or frozen)
- 2 tablespoons chopped nuts (almonds, walnuts, or pecans)

Instructions:

1. In a jar or container with a tight-fitting lid, combine the oats, almond milk, yogurt, chia seeds, and vanilla extract. Stir well to combine.
2. Cover and refrigerate overnight, or for at least 4 hours.
3. When ready to serve, top with berries and chopped nuts. Enjoy cold or at room temperature.

Nutrition per serving: 350 calories, 14g protein, 44g carbohydrates, 11g fiber, 14g fat, 1.5g saturated fat, 0mg cholesterol, 65mg sodium.

Tips: Use a variety of different berries and nuts to keep things interesting, and feel free to adjust the ratio of oats to liquid to achieve your desired consistency. For an extra heart-healthy boost, add a tablespoon of ground flaxseed or a sprinkle of cinnamon.

2. Avocado and White Bean Toast
Ingredients:
- 2 slices whole-grain bread, toasted
- 1/2 ripe avocado, mashed
- 1/4 cup canned white beans, rinsed and drained

- 1 tablespoon lemon juice
- 1/4 teaspoon garlic powder
- 1/4 teaspoon salt
- 1/4 teaspoon black pepper
- 1/4 cup sliced cherry tomatoes
- 2 tablespoons chopped fresh basil

Instructions:

1. In a small bowl, combine the mashed avocado, white beans, lemon juice, garlic powder, salt, and black pepper. Mix well.
2. Spread the avocado mixture evenly over the toasted bread slices.
3. Top with sliced cherry tomatoes and fresh basil. Serve immediately.

Nutrition per serving: 320 calories, 11g protein, 39g carbohydrates, 11g fiber, 16g fat, 2g saturated fat, 0mg cholesterol, 520mg sodium.

Tips: For a spicier kick, add a pinch of red pepper flakes to the avocado mixture. You can also experiment with different types of beans, such as chickpeas or black beans, for variety.

Lunches
1. Mediterranean Quinoa Salad
Ingredients:
- 1 cup uncooked quinoa, rinsed
- 2 cups water
- 1/2 cup cherry tomatoes, halved
- 1/2 cup cucumber, diced
- 1/4 cup red onion, diced
- 1/4 cup Kalamata olives, pitted and halved
- 1/4 cup crumbled feta cheese
- 2 tablespoons chopped fresh parsley

- 2 tablespoons lemon juice
- 1 tablespoon extra-virgin olive oil
- 1/4 teaspoon salt
- 1/4 teaspoon black pepper

Instructions:

1. In a medium saucepan, bring the quinoa and water to a boil. Reduce heat to low, cover, and simmer for 15 minutes, or until the water is absorbed and the quinoa is tender.
2. Remove from heat and let stand, covered, for 5 minutes. Fluff with a fork and transfer to a large bowl.
3. Add the tomatoes, cucumber, onion, olives, feta, and parsley to the quinoa. Toss gently to combine.
4. In a small bowl, whisk together the lemon juice, olive oil, salt, and black pepper. Pour over the quinoa mixture and toss to coat.
5. Serve warm or at room temperature.

Nutrition per serving: 320 calories, 10g protein, 42g carbohydrates, 5g fiber, 12g fat, 3g saturated fat, 10mg cholesterol, 370mg sodium.

Tips: For a vegan version, omit the feta cheese or replace it with a plant-based alternative. You can also add other Mediterranean-inspired ingredients, such as roasted red peppers or artichoke hearts, for extra flavor and nutrition.

2. Spicy Black Bean Wraps
   Ingredients:
   - 4 whole-grain tortillas
   - 1 can (15 ounces) black beans, rinsed and drained
   - 1/2 cup salsa
   - 1/2 teaspoon cumin
   - 1/2 teaspoon chili powder

- 1/4 teaspoon garlic powder
- 1/2 cup shredded lettuce
- 1/2 cup diced tomatoes
- 1/4 cup diced red onion
- 1/4 cup chopped fresh cilantro

Instructions:

1. In a medium bowl, mash the black beans with a fork or potato masher. Stir in the salsa, cumin, chili powder, and garlic powder.
2. Warm the tortillas in the microwave or on a griddle until pliable.
3. Divide the bean mixture evenly among the tortillas, spreading it in a line down the center of each one.
4. Top with lettuce, tomatoes, onion, and cilantro.
5. Roll up the tortillas tightly, tucking in the ends as you go. Slice in half diagonally and serve.

Nutrition per serving: 280 calories, 12g protein, 48g carbohydrates, 12g fiber, 4g fat, 0g saturated fat, 0mg cholesterol, 600mg sodium.

Tips: Experiment with different types of salsa, such as roasted tomato or tomatillo, for variety. You can also add other veggies, such as bell peppers or corn, for extra crunch and nutrition.

Dinners
1. Baked Salmon with Lemon and Dill
Ingredients:
- 4 salmon fillets (4 ounces each)
- 1 tablespoon extra-virgin olive oil
- 1/2 teaspoon salt
- 1/4 teaspoon black pepper
- 1 lemon, thinly sliced

- 4 sprigs fresh dill
- Lemon wedges, for serving

Instructions:

1. Preheat the oven to 400°F (200°C).
2. Place the salmon fillets in a baking dish. Drizzle with olive oil and sprinkle with salt and pepper.
3. Arrange the lemon slices and dill sprigs over the salmon.
4. Bake for 12-15 minutes, or until the salmon is cooked through and flakes easily with a fork.
5. Serve hot, with lemon wedges on the side.

Nutrition per serving: 220 calories, 24g protein, 1g carbohydrates, 0g fiber, 12g fat, 2g saturated fat, 60mg cholesterol, 350mg sodium.

Tips: For a complete meal, serve the salmon with steamed vegetables and quinoa or brown rice. You can also experiment with different herbs and spices, such as rosemary or garlic, for variety.

2. Vegetarian Chili
Ingredients:
- 1 tablespoon extra-virgin olive oil
- 1 onion, diced
- 2 cloves garlic, minced
- 1 red bell pepper, diced
- 1 can (15 ounces) black beans, rinsed and drained
- 1 can (15 ounces) kidney beans, rinsed and drained
- 1 can (14.5 ounces) diced tomatoes, with juice
- 1 cup vegetable broth
- 1 tablespoon chili powder
- 1 teaspoon ground cumin

- 1/2 teaspoon smoked paprika
- 1/4 teaspoon salt
- 1/4 teaspoon black pepper
- 1/4 cup chopped fresh cilantro

Instructions:

1. In a large pot or Dutch oven, heat the olive oil over medium heat. Add the onion, garlic, and bell pepper, and cook until softened, about 5 minutes.
2. Add the black beans, kidney beans, tomatoes, vegetable broth, chili powder, cumin, smoked paprika, salt, and black pepper. Stir to combine.
3. Bring to a boil, then reduce heat and simmer for 20-25 minutes, or until the flavors have melded and the chili has thickened slightly.
4. Serve hot, garnished with fresh cilantro.

Nutrition per serving: 250 calories, 12g protein, 41g carbohydrates, 13g fiber, 5g fat, 1g saturated fat, 0mg cholesterol, 600mg sodium.

Tips: For a heartier meal, serve the chili over brown rice or with whole-grain cornbread. You can also top it with diced avocado, shredded cheese, or a dollop of plain Greek yogurt for extra flavor and nutrition.

Snacks and Desserts
1. Roasted Chickpeas
Ingredients:
- 1 can (15 ounces) chickpeas, rinsed, drained, and patted dry
- 1 tablespoon extra-virgin olive oil
- 1/2 teaspoon garlic powder
- 1/2 teaspoon smoked paprika
- 1/4 teaspoon salt
- 1/4 teaspoon black pepper

Instructions:

1. Preheat the oven to 400°F (200°C).
2. In a bowl, toss the chickpeas with the olive oil, garlic powder, smoked paprika, salt, and black pepper.
3. Spread the chickpeas in a single layer on a baking sheet.
4. Roast for 30-40 minutes, stirring occasionally, until the chickpeas are crispy and golden brown.
5. Let cool for 5-10 minutes before serving.

Nutrition per serving: 120 calories, 5g protein, 16g carbohydrates, 5g fiber, 5g fat, 0.5g saturated fat, 0mg cholesterol, 200mg sodium.

Tips: Experiment with different spice blends, such as curry powder or Italian seasoning, for variety. Roasted chickpeas make a great snack on their own, or you can use them as a crunchy topping for salads or soups.

2. Chocolate Avocado Mousse
   Ingredients:
   - 2 ripe avocados, pitted and peeled
   - 1/2 cup unsweetened cocoa powder
   - 1/2 cup pure maple syrup
   - 1/4 cup unsweetened almond milk
   - 1 teaspoon vanilla extract
   - Pinch of salt
   - Fresh berries, for serving

Instructions:

1. In a food processor or blender, combine the avocados, cocoa powder, maple syrup, almond milk, vanilla extract, and salt. Process until smooth and creamy, scraping down the sides as needed.

2. Transfer the mousse to individual serving dishes and refrigerate for at least 30 minutes, or until chilled.
3. Serve topped with fresh berries.

Nutrition per serving: 230 calories, 4g protein, 33g carbohydrates, 10g fiber, 12g fat, 2g saturated fat, 0mg cholesterol, 25mg sodium.

Tips: For a richer, more decadent mousse, use full-fat coconut milk instead of almond milk. You can also experiment with different toppings, such as chopped nuts or shredded coconut, for variety.

Conclusion

Eating for heart health doesn't have to be boring or restrictive. With a little creativity and inspiration, you can enjoy a wide variety of delicious, nutritious meals that support healthy cholesterol levels and overall cardiovascular well-being.

The recipes in this chapter are just a starting point – a way to showcase the principles of heart-healthy eating in action. Use them as a foundation for your own culinary explorations, experimenting with different ingredients, flavors, and techniques to create meals that nourish your body and delight your senses.

Remember, the key to sustainable, enjoyable eating habits is to focus on whole, minimally processed foods, with an emphasis on plant-based ingredients like fruits, vegetables, whole grains, legumes, nuts, and seeds. By filling your plate with these nutrient-dense foods, you'll be well on your way to a heart-healthy life – one delicious bite at a time.

So go ahead and get cooking! With a little kitchen magic and a lot of love, you can create a meal plan that supports your cholesterol goals, satisfies your cravings, and leaves you feeling nourished, energized, and inspired. Your heart (and your taste buds) will thank you.

CONCLUSION

Conclusion: Embracing a Heart-Healthy Lifestyle for Lifelong Wellness

Throughout this book, we've explored the many facets of lowering cholesterol naturally and promoting overall heart health. From understanding the role of cholesterol in the body to adopting a nutrient-rich, plant-forward diet, incorporating regular exercise and stress management techniques, and partnering with healthcare providers for personalized guidance and support, we've covered a wide range of strategies for optimizing cardiovascular wellness.

At the heart of all of these strategies is a simple but powerful truth: that the choices we make each day – the foods we eat, the activities we engage in, the thoughts we think, and the habits we cultivate – have a profound impact on our health and well-being. By making small, consistent changes in these areas, we can create a ripple effect of positive transformation that extends far beyond our cholesterol levels alone.

Embracing a heart-healthy lifestyle is not about achieving perfection or adhering to a rigid set of rules. Rather, it's about developing a mindset of self-care and self-compassion, and making choices that honor our bodies, minds, and spirits. It's about nourishing ourselves with whole, natural foods that provide the building blocks for optimal health, engaging in activities that bring us joy and fulfillment, and cultivating relationships and practices that support our emotional and spiritual well-being.

This holistic approach to heart health recognizes that true wellness is not just about the absence of disease, but about the presence of vitality, resilience, and joy. It acknowledges that our physical, mental, and emotional health are intricately interconnected, and that by tending to each of these areas with care and intention, we can create a foundation of well-being that sustains us throughout our lives.

Of course, making lasting changes to our lifestyle habits is not always easy. It requires patience, persistence, and a willingness to learn from our setbacks and celebrate our successes along the way. It may involve challenging long-held beliefs and patterns of behavior, and stepping outside of our comfort zones to try new things. But with the right tools, support, and mindset, it is possible to transform our health and our lives in profound and lasting ways.

One of the most empowering aspects of adopting a heart-healthy lifestyle is the realization that we are the authors of our own health stories. While we may not have control over every factor that influences our cardiovascular health, such as genetics or certain environmental exposures, we do have the power to make choices each day that support our well-being and reduce our risk of chronic disease.

By taking a proactive, engaged approach to our health – by educating ourselves about the factors that influence our cholesterol levels and overall cardiovascular wellness, by partnering with trusted healthcare providers to develop personalized prevention and treatment plans, and by making consistent, intentional choices that align with our values and goals – we can become the heroes of our own health journeys.

This process of empowerment and self-discovery is not a one-time event, but a lifelong journey of growth and learning. As we deepen our understanding of what truly nourishes and sustains us, we may find that our definitions of health and happiness evolve over time. What once seemed like a sacrifice or a chore – such as giving up certain foods or committing to regular exercise – may become a source of joy and vitality, an integral part of our daily lives.

As we've seen throughout this book, there is no one-size-fits-all approach to lowering cholesterol and promoting heart health. Each person's journey will be unique, shaped by their individual needs, preferences, and life circumstances. What works for one person may not work for another, and what feels sustainable and enjoyable at one stage of life may need to be adapted as our bodies and priorities change.

The key is to remain curious, open-minded, and compassionate with ourselves and others as we navigate this journey. To seek out reliable information and guidance from trusted sources, while also tuning in to our own inner wisdom and intuition. To surround ourselves with people and practices that uplift and inspire us, and to let go of those that no longer serve our highest good.

As we come to the end of this book, it is my hope that you feel empowered and inspired to take charge of your own heart health story. That you have gained valuable insights and practical strategies for lowering your cholesterol naturally, reducing your risk of cardiovascular disease, and enhancing your overall well-being. And that you feel supported and motivated to continue learning, growing, and thriving on your personal path to lifelong wellness.

Remember, the journey of a thousand miles begins with a single step. Every choice you make – whether it's to enjoy a colorful, plant-based meal, to go for a heartening walk in nature, to practice a few minutes of mindful breathing, or to reach out for support when you need it – is a step in the right direction. A step towards greater health, happiness, and wholeness.

So keep taking those steps, one day at a time. Celebrate your progress, learn from your setbacks, and trust in your own resilience and capacity for positive change. Surround yourself with people and practices that nourish and uplift you, and let go of those that no longer serve your highest good.

And above all, remember that you are the author of your own health story. You have the power to shape your life and your well-being in ways that are truly authentic and meaningful to you. So embrace that power, and use it to create a heart-healthy life that fills you with vitality, joy, and purpose.

On behalf of myself and the entire team behind this book, I wish you all the best on your journey to lifelong heart health and happiness. May you find the strength, wisdom, and support you need to thrive, and may you always know that you are deserving of a life filled with love, laughter, and optimal well-being.